AF677090

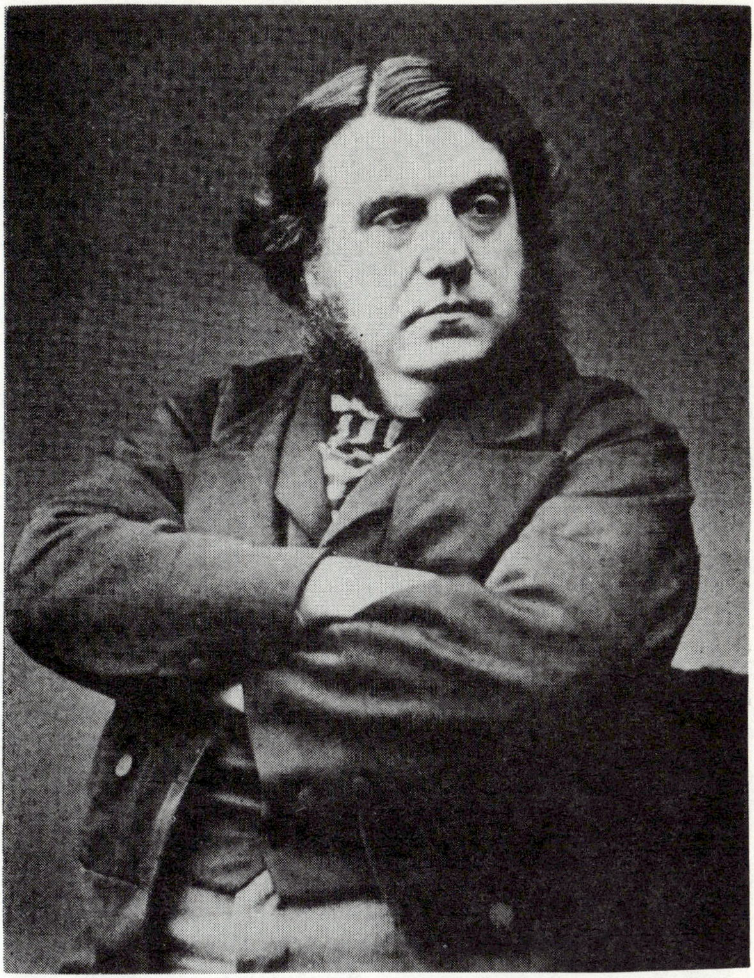

I Robert Lawson Tait (1845-1899)

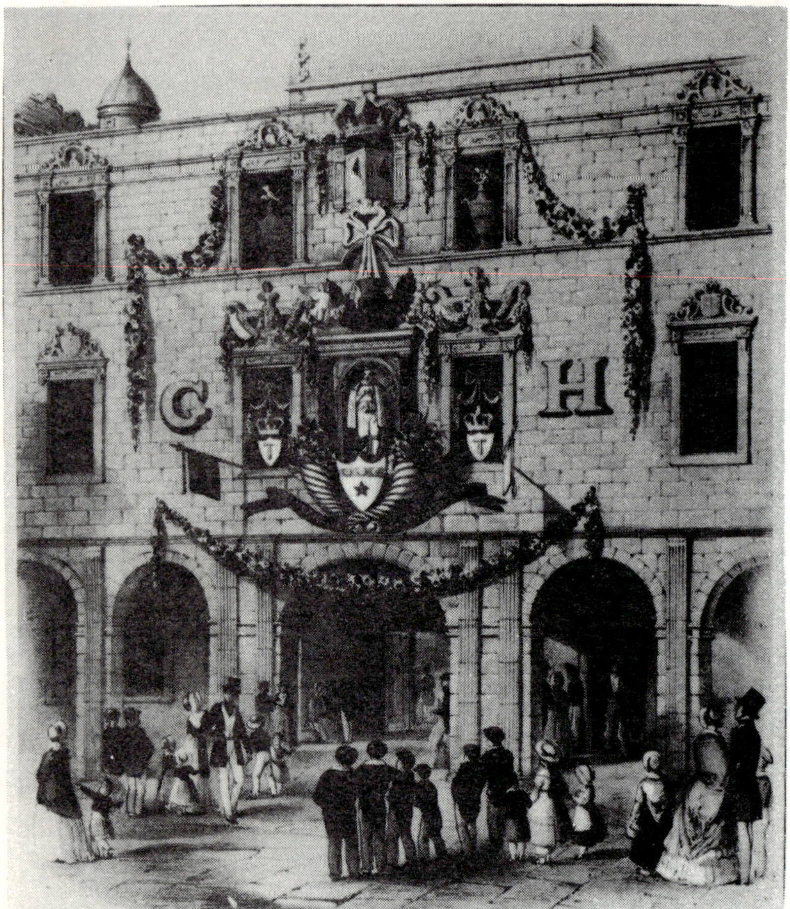

II Bicentenary celebrations at George Heriots School
in 1859, when Tait was a pupil
(By permission of Edinburgh City Library)

LAWSON TAIT
THE REBELLIOUS SURGEON
(1845-1899)

by
John A. Shepherd

Coronado Press 1980

ISBN 0–87291–131–4

Set in 10 on twelve point Press Roman
and published in the United States of America
by Coronado Press: Box 3232, Lawrence, Kansas
66044

CONTENTS

LIST OF ILLUSTRATIONS

At End

Lawson Tait
The Rebellious Surgeon

PREFACE

In any history of the evolution of surgery in the 19th century Joseph Lister must be predominant for his introduction of antisepsis. There were many others, however, who made significant advances, among them Robert Lawson Tait. He began his surgical career in 1867, the year in which Lister's work was first published. He was involved at the beginning of the great controversy concerning Listerism, a controversy largely initiated by Simpson of Edinburgh. The young Tait, an ardent disciple of Simpson, soon became antagonistic to Lister's teaching. Tait's arguments were sometimes illogical and perhaps partisan in origin but a study of his interventions in this debate brings greater understanding of the reluctance with which Lister's work was accepted in Great Britain. Tait's critical attitude was not unproductive, for he shares some credit for the fairly rapid transition from antiseptic to aseptic principles in surgery.

Tait exerted great influence in many other directions and in a space of fifteen years he rose to a position of authority and eminence. In his later years, for a variety of reasons, his reputation declined and so when he died many of his achievements were forgotten.

My interest in Tait was aroused many years ago when I had occasion to do some research into the history of the surgery of the acute abdomen. I soon discovered that he was one of the pioneers in both acute and elective abdominal surgery. I read the biography published in 1922 by his Australian pupil, Stewart McKay, and was fascinated by Tait's energy, originality and unusual character. Both in McKay's account and in a later one by Harvey Flack, I felt there were gaps in the story and that there was room for a more critical and complete appraisal of the life and work of Lawson Tait.

Tait was greatly influenced by his Edinburgh training and my study of two of his teachers, Simpson and Syme, has helped me to understand Tait's surgical philosophy. The preparation of a biography of one of Tait's contemporaries, Thomas Spencer Wells, has also aided me. Wells was the antithesis of Tait in his professional and social life and it was inevitable that the brash young provincial should clash with the older, domineering leader of the conservative London Establishment. The bitter feud between these two surgeons reflects the jealous professional rivalries of the Victorian age. Such vendettas had considerable influence on Tait's attitudes.

In his brief and at times stormy career Tait contributed basic concepts of surgery still held today, but he was responsible also for many new and important technical innovations and operative procedures. I believe that his surgical achievements have not been fully recognised and that it is now possible to evaluate them more completely.

While Tait was not alone amongst Victorian doctors in his participation in affairs outside his professional life, there were few who devoted such energy to so many additional projects and causes. His association with Charles Darwin, for example, is of special interest. Few other clinicians recognised the significance of the new theory of evolution to medical science. Such episodes in Tait's life make his story all the more intriguing and reveal his complex personality in such a way that there must be admiration for his virtues and achievements and sympathy and understanding for his foibles and failures.

I have drawn freely on the earlier biographies but wherever possible I have checked such details as have been derived from these. The medical press of Tait's period abounds with references to his movements, for he was always "news". His own writings, whether on surgical or on unrelated topics, provide much autobiographical information. No large collections of letters or other private papers have been traced with the exception of the Darwin correspondence.

It is impossible to list all of the many colleagues and friends who have given encouragement, criticism or information. Those who have encouraged me include Professor Owen Wangensteen and the late Sir Zachary Cope. Dr. Bryn Thomas generously read and criticised the completed text. Dr. Frank Forster and Sir Edward Ford of Melbourne put me on the track of unpublished autobiographical material concerning Tait and written by McKay. Dr. Sydney Smith introduced me to the Darwin collection in the Cambridge University Library, in which are preserved Tait's letters to Darwin. Dr. Smith very kindly read the script of Chapter VII and clarified for me some of the more abstruse aspects of Darwinism. Through the good offices of Surgeon Rear Admiral Cyril McLintock I was put in touch with Mrs. Ernestine Phillips, who has in her possession many relics of Tait and some important letters. She very generously has allowed me to make use of this valuable material. Dr. F. T. Davis was very helpful in locating for me various documents having reference to Tait's Birmingham connections. Others who very kindly sent me information of great value were Sir Hedley Atkins, Mr. Eagar,

Dr. W. B. Gough and Mr. A. Maxwell Reader. Dr. O'Brien very kindly showed me the stable where Tait had a laboratory, behind Westfield house in Wakefield. Mrs. Lea took me over St. Petrocks, near Llandudno, the house in which Tait died. Mr. Hugh Stewart, a descendant of the family of Tait's wife told me something of his forebears.

The medical historian depends greatly on librarians for help, which is always given most generously. I must thank, in particular, Mr. Crook (and before him, the late Mr. Lee) of the Liverpool Medical Institution, Mr. Sutherland of the British Medical Association Library, Mr. Taylor of the Birmingham City Library, Miss Wardle of the Library of the Royal College of Surgeons of Edinburgh and Mr. Willox of the Wakefield City Library.

Acknowledgement of permission to publish certain plates is made in the list of illustrations (above, page viii). For permission to print extracts of Tait's letters to Charles Darwin I must thank the Syndics of the University Library, Cambridge. The Chairman and Governors of Shrewsbury School have allowed me to quote from the Darwin letters in their possession.The Editors of the Lancet and the British Medical Journal have permitted me to quote freely from their publications.

Professor Wangensteen put me in touch with Professor John Longhurst and the Coronado Press. Any misgivings I may have had concerning problems of distance soon evaporated. Professor Longhurst and his staff could not have been more helpful in the preparation of this book which will, I hope, be of interest to readers in The United States as well as in Great Britain. Finally, I am much indebted to Mrs. Ella Henderson for her patient and expert preparation of the typescript.

John Shepherd
Liverpool, England

CHAPTER I

Origins and Upbringing (1845-1867)

It is tempting to ascribe to parents or earlier forebears the genes of intelligence, character and temperament. Such attributions may have a scientific basis or may be fanciful. A biographer may try to evaluate also the influence of the early environment and education on his subject, thus to explain behaviour, to account for virtues and, sometimes, to condone defects.

For Robert Lawson Tait the material available concerning such influences is sparse. It may be for this reason that his first biographer, Stewart McKay, accepted some unproven statements and presented these as established facts which in subsequent years have seldom been refuted.[1] McKay maintained that Lawson Tait was the son of an Edinburgh lawyer or Writer to the Signet who was cousin to the distinguished churchman Campbell Tait, Archbishop of Canterbury from 1868 to 1882. Doubtless McKay copied this information from obituaries written on Tait's death in 1899. It is difficult to understand why this inaccuracy was not questioned at the time. Such an origin would imply that, born into a professional family, Lawson Tait would have had certain advantages. Few problems concerning education, professional advancement or social acceptance would have been presented when, at this time, entry into a learned profession was certainly easier for the well-connected than for those of humble birth.

There are many examples of notable figures in medicine in the 19th century who, despite disadvantages of birth, rose to great fame. Sir James Young Simpson, the son of an impoverished baker in a small Scottish town, springs to mind. He rose to great distinction supported, in the Scottish tradition, by his brothers and sisters who sacrificed much so that the young hopeful in the family could have the opportunities of a university education. Lawson Tait was, like Simpson, of humble origin. By recognising this we may understand his character much more clearly, his faults as well as his virtues and, in particular, his attitudes to his professional contemporaries. He lived in an age in which the barriers of class were more significant in determining social acceptance and professional success than pertains today.

That he was born in Edinburgh is reasonably certain. There is no confirmation of his birth from registration, for this was not compulsory in Scotland until 1855. Alternative proof by certification of baptism has not been traced; indeed the religion of his parents is uncertain although it is said he was born into the Roman Catholic faith. There is a fair supposition that he was born on May 1, 1845. McKay specifies 45 Frederick Street, Edinburgh as the birthplace.[2] In 1845 his father is not recorded in the contemporary Edinburgh directory as a householder at that address but several families are listed as occupants and perhaps the Tait family lodged there.

His father was Archibald Campbell Tait. This is confirmed by the inscription on the tombstone of his mother and by entries in the records of George Heriot's School where Lawson Tait was enrolled in 1852.[3] Little is known of Archibald Tait; we do know that he came to Edinburgh from Drymen in Stirlingshire. His occupation is recorded variously as "vintner" and "butler" in the Heriot's School records. In the Edinburgh Directory of 1839 he appears as a vintner living in the Fleshmarket Close and he is included in the list of Burghers and Guild brothers of that year. This implies that he was then a householder. In subsequent years his name disappears from the Directories except that in 1850 one Archibald Tait, whose occupation is not stated, is recorded as lodging in a house in Princes Street. It must be surmised that soon after 1839 his circumstances deteriorated and he may well have run into financial difficulties. There is some evidence that Archibald Tait died when his son was a medical student.

Tait's mother was Isabella Stewart Lawson, a native of Leven in Fife, but the year of her marriage is not known. As a widow she went to live with her son when he became established as a surgeon in Birmingham and there she died in 1882. She had two other sons whose names are recorded on her tombstone, both of whom died in childhood.[4]

From such limited information it would appear that Tait's upbringing was relatively humble and perhaps at times in conditions near poverty. Nevertheless a pleasing photograph of a studious, well-nourished, well-clad little boy of 11 survives to suggest that there were bright periods in his childhood. It is recorded that his mother was irascible in her old age; however, there was devotion between mother and son, demonstrated by the way Tait cared for his mother to the end of her days. Lawson tait made no pretensions about his origins and described his parents as "perfectly respectable, if not distinguished".[5]

He must have shown unusual intelligence and promise at an early age, for he was accepted as a foundation scholar in George Heriot's School in October 1852. That his father had been a burgess of the city, fallen perhaps on hard times, would have facilitated the boy's acceptance as a bursar.

This well-known Edinburgh school was founded in the 17th century by the benefaction of George Heriot, a jeweller and goldsmith who flourished in the time of James VI. Heriot was jeweller to the Court in London and in his will he left part of his considerable fortune to erect a hospital in the city of Edinburgh for the "maintenance, relief, bringing up and education. . . . of so many poor fatherless boys, freemans' sons of the town of Edinburgh". Originally there was provision for only 10 Bursars but as the years passed the school expanded. In 1834 it provided for "burgesses' bairns, and their parents not able to maintain them". The education afforded was of a high quality with instruction in the classics, in mathematics and in scientific subjects. In 1855 there was even a course of lectures on physiology given by a Dr. Hodgson. The school, by the mid-19th century, had nurtured many who made their names in the legal and the medical professions. A bias towards medicine may have been related to the appointments as surgeons to the school of William Wood and then his son Andrew Wood, successively Presidents of the Royal College of Surgeons of Edinburgh.

Robert Tait is recorded as a "house bursar" in 1859 and presumably on entry he held some form of foundation bursary i.e., ascholarship). In a history of the school published in 1859 there is a long account of the celebrations in that year of the bicentenary of its foundation, at which event Tait must have been present. There is also in this history a glossary of the vernacular spoken by the boys and there is an imaginary, and almost incomprehensible, dialogue between two of them, one being recorded as "Tait". This may have been Lawson Tait; if so, the conversation must be regarded as his first published utterances. It is a curious point that in the many detailed descriptions of him there is no suggestion that a Scottish accent survived into adult life.[6]

Lawson Tait must have done well at school, but the only report which can be traced is of July 1859 and reads: "Headmaster's estimate of talent: very good scholar: Bursar: generally well behaved: hopeful scholar". His progress was certainly sufficient to ensure matriculation at Edinburgh University on November 1, 1859. He was then aged 14 and a half years but at the time it was not unusual to enter University so young. Initially he enrolled in the Faculty of Arts but in his second and third years he is entered in the lists of the Faculty of Medicine. In these three years he does not appear in any University prize list. However, after qualification he recorded in the Medical Directory that he was "First Prizeman in Surgery at the College in Edinburgh". This distinction he must have gained after the autumn of 1862 when he transferred to the Extramural School of Medicine there to complete his medical training.

By 1855 the Extramural School had been recognised officially by the University and it was permissible for matriculated students to attend up to half of their classes there. Extramural teaching in Edinburgh had flourished greatly despite the rival attraction of an university course of medical education of international renown. The long survival and the popularity of the extramural school, despite initial antagonism from the University, was related very largely to the brilliance of such teachers as John Bell, Charles Bell, Lizars, Barclay, Knox and Liston (in anatomy and surgery), Sharpey (in physiology), Wood (in medicine), and Thatcher and Simpson (in midwifery). To some degree the quality of teaching in certain university departments had declined after 1830. For example, the contribution of Professor Monro, the third of his line in the Chair of Anatomy, scarcely equalled that of the extramural anatomical teachers.[7]

Lawson Tait's move from the University to the Extramural School is not readily explained, but this was not unusual for students at this period. In 1862 there was sufficient agreement between the two teaching bodies to allow such a change without detriment to qualification. It is possible that fees were less in the Extramural School; this, when Tait's mother was widowed and most likely very poor, may have been significant. It is not impossible that Tait fell afoul of one or other of the University Professors as at an early stage he showed some aggressive qualities and perhaps tended to criticise his elders in an outspoken fashion. A photograph of him as a student reveals a very determined young man.

Of those whose influence Tait acknowledged in later years, some were in the University and some in the Extramural School. While much instruction was given by the didactic lecture, there was still a survival, if unofficial, of the apprentice system by which a student worked very closely with his teacher and assisted him in both hospital and private practice. Lawson Tait recorded that for five years he had been "apprentice, pupil and assistant" to the surgeon Alexander McKenzie Edwards (? -1868), but he was probably merely a dresser in Edwards' wards at different stages of his student career. It is unlikely that he paid Edwards a fee, although this practice did continue sporadically up to 1862. Tait often recalled Edwards' teaching with gratitude. Edwards was not a very well-known surgeon, but as a young man he showed great promise as a pupil of William Fergusson. He was a lecturer in surgery in the Extramural School from 1859 and he died comparatively young.

Of other teachers to whom Tait owed inspiration or encouragement there were, in particular, Littlejohn, Syme, and Simpson.

Dr. Littlejohn, later Professor Sir Henry Littlejohn (1826-1914), became Extramural lecturer in Medical Jurisprudence in 1855. He was an exceptional teacher who attracted huge classes. Appointed the first medical officer of health in Edinburgh in 1862, he was a pioneer, with Sir Edwin Chadwick (1800-1890), of sanitary science. Littlejohn's activities brought down dramatically the appalling death rate from disease in the teeming slums of the old town of Edinburgh and he may well have aroused in the mind of a receptive student like Lawson Tait an interest in the problems of public health and in the control of infection.

Professor James Syme (1799-1870) was at the peak of his career in 1860, the acknowledged master of surgery in Scotland and recognised internationally. Terse, dogmatic, conservative, and at times unapproachable to many, he was to intimate friends a sympathetic, kindly man, consistent and honest in all his activities and dedicated to surgery and its teaching. Lawson Tait often recalled Syme's operative ability, his careful and clean technique and his simple but able teaching. It does not appear that Tait had any close contact with Syme, but like most Edinburgh students, he respected him greatly and fell under his spell. In 1860 Syme's brilliant protégé Joseph Lister (1827-1912) had gone to Glasgow as Professor of Surgery, but he often revisited Edinburgh to assist Syme in major operations. Lister returned to Edinburgh to succeed Syme in the Chair of Clinical Surgery in 1869, but by this date Tait had gone to England. There is no indication that Tait as a student met Lister, but he must have heard of his activities in Glasgow and he saw him assist Syme in at least one dramatic operation. Tait was to become one of Lister's most vociferous critics.

James Young Simpson (1811-1870) too was at the peak of his career about 1860, holding the Chair of Midwifery. He was the most dynamic and original of the Edinburgh professors, famed for his pioneer work on anaesthesia culminating in the discovery of the use of chloroform. He was recognised internationally as an authority on obstetrics and gynaecology. With his extraordinary versatility his interests ranged through all the branches of medicine and surgery. At an early stage Tait became known to Simpson and often recounted how closely he had worked as a student with the great obstetrician. Like other students, he lived for short spells at 52 Queen's Street in the Simpson household, while acting as a student assistant. He often referred to operations at which he had assisted Simpson, to specimens dissected for him and he followed closely all his multifarious interests and activities.[8]

In 1858 Simpson first described his method of the control of bleeding by acupressure and in 1864 he published a large monograph on the subject.[9] He believed that the orthodox method of ligation of blood vessels with thread or other materials induced poor healing or even fatal effects. He proposed instead that blood vessels should be controlled by under-running them with long pins or needles which were retained for one or two days until the pressure so applied had sealed off the flattened vessel. He was convinced that this new technique would prove revolutionary. Despite some acceptance by a few contemporary surgeons acupressure was a failure and any hope of its general acceptance was swept away by the presentation by Lister, in 1867, of his concept of antiseptic surgery. Lister's work established the fact that the ligature could be used without the risk of inducing infection of wounds.

As a student Lawson Tait was involved directly in Simpson's abortive but nevertheless significant research on haemostasis by acupressure and in 1865 he published an article in the *Medical Times and Gazette,* "On the results of temporary metallic compression of arteries". He reported a series of 28 experiments on cats and dogs by which he showed how acupressure worked. Simpson apparently suggested these experiments so that he might refute the theories of Professor Weber (probably Ernst Weber [1795-1878]), a distinguished anatomist and physiologist of Leipzig). Weber believed that acupressure caused gangrene of blood vessels by compression, while Simpson believed that control of bleeding was achieved without such severe effects, but by simple adhesion of the inner wall of a vessel, aided occasionally by thrombosis within its lumen. Tait's carefully documented experiments supported Simpson's explanation. The work took six months and was done in the laboratory of Dr. Gamgee (probably in the Veterinary College).[10] As well as describing these animal experiments Tait discussed the practical lessons he had learnt and illustrated his arguments from dissections of material from Simpson's practice.

That an unqualified young student should have conducted such a painstaking series of animal experiments and should then have had his report published, refuting the opinions of an influential foreign professor, was unusual, but Tait was an unusual student.

Soon after he qualified Tait wrote descriptions of his methods of preparing and mounting pathological specimens and he indicated that he had been accumulating his own museum from the time he was a second year student. There are many references in his subsequent writings to cases he saw while a student, specimens he dissected and mounted, operations at which he assisted and autopsies he performed. He was original, industrious, and enthusiastic.

Tait's relationship with Simpson requires further comment. It is uncertain just how definite was his attachment to Simpson as an assistant, but his experimental project does suggest a close association. The young student admired Simpson from the first and his admiration never flagged. Tait was to champion many of Simpson's causes long after "his master" died. For his part, Simpson recognised that here was an exceptional young man worthy of encouragement.

But another explanation has been advanced of Simpson's interest in Lawson Tait. To this day there are some who believe that he was a natural son of Simpson. If this were true, then in any attempt to assess Tait's character and achievement we cannot ignore the potential repercussions of the stigma of illegitimacy or the possible psychological effects.

It is difficult to discover when this allegation was first made. McKay, in an unpublished manuscript of an autobiography, describes how when he was Tait's assistant in Birmingham, finding him in an expansive mood during a holiday weekend, he asked him to describe Simpson's appearance. McKay writes:[11]

> Tait immediately turned and looked at me, then he seemed to change his mind for he took off his hat, pulled down some of his long hair over the side of his forehead and ears and said, "There, now you see him: they say I am his illegitimate son. . . ."

Until this incident, which must have been about 1891, McKay had not heard even a rumour of such a relationship. He records, however, that when he later visited Edinburgh he was told by more than one medical man that there was no doubt about Simpson being Tait's father and that the mother was a woman of title. Soon after Tait's death in 1899, the Simpson family found it necessary to deny the rumour by a letter to the public press. It is possible that the story got around even in Simpson's lifetime.

In his biography of Tait, McKay places portraits of each alongside, alleging a strong physical resemblance. Certainly both had massive heads, but the features and hands are not very similar. On account of physical resemblance, McKay attributed much of Tait's character to direct inheritance trom Simpson.

In 1844, the year before Lawson Tait was born, Simpson was a rising young professor, happily married and with three children. His first child, a girl, died in that year at the age of four. There are many letters extant which reveal Simpson's great grief at this event. It is not impossible, but somewhat unlikely, that Simpson should have been unfaithful to his wife at such a time. In his lifetime Simpson did not escape accusations of immorality. A book entitled *Stories of the Temple in Edinburgh* was published anonymously in 1862 (but its distribution was quickly suppressed). This was a virulent attack on Simpson, imputing immoral behaviour in his medical practice. It was rather typical of the slanderous publications appearing in professional circles in the mid-Victorian period, arising either from intense professional jealousy or perhaps from perverted minds. Before this particular attack was published Simpson had been accused by the wife of his secretary of being the father of a child which Simpson had fostered out to her. This charge, which was eventually made public, much to Simpson's detriment, was almost certainly false; it emanated from a woman who, from her letters, seems clearly to have been mentally deranged. She was obsessed with the idea that Simpson had dismissed her husband from his service unfairly and thereby ruined his career.[12]

If Lawson Tait was Simpson's illegitimate son it seems unlikely that he would have been brought into the household when he was a student. If, as some have suggested, Simpson did take a special interest in Tait because he was in fact his illegitimate son, then why did he not help in his earlier education? There is no evidence that he did so. On balance the case is not convincing, but Tait may well have encouraged the rumour, for he was not averse to startling or shocking his friends. There are no comments which he himself made about his early life which suggest that he really believed that Archibald and Isabella Tait were not his lawful parents.

The undoubted resemblances of character and the common interests of Simpson and Tait can be readily explained by the hero worship of a student for his chief. This is not so very uncommon; sometimes it is transitory, but sometimes it lasts for life. Thus, by imitation, Tait developed some of Simpson's mannerisms; he showed the same intense industry, he had the same enthusiasm for anything new (and sometimes the tendency to jump too rapidly to conclusions), and the same love of argument. Both men had a curiosity which extended not only to branches of medicine outside their specialities but also to other sciences, to archaeology, and many other fields. Tait, at the start of his career, appeared to model his style on Simpson.

It is curious that in the large collection of letters hoarded by Simpson, of those which survive none is from Tait in the four years after he qualified up to Simpson's death in 1870.[13] It seems most unlikely that they did not correspond in this period, for both were inveterate letter writers. It is possible, however, that the family, who after Simpson's death were very much aware of a wave of accusations against his character and of the suggestion of Tait's illegitimate relationship, destroyed such letters to dissociate him as completely as possible.

Tait was among the select few who, on the occasion of Simpson's funeral, was admitted to the house as a family friend. He was asked by the family to complete some unfinished papers by Simpson. Finally, it is fascinating to find that six years after Tait died in 1899 his ashes were buried in Warriston Cemetery not far from Simpson's grave. This must surely have been because of a wish expressed by Tait before he died and can be seen as an indication of Tait's adulation of Simpson, and nothing more. Throughout his life, Tait never ceased to express his gratitude to one who had recognised his early promise, taught him well, given him special opportunities, and set him on the path to success.[14]

Before Tait published his work on acupressure in 1865 a communication from him was read at a meeting of the Obstetrical Society of Edinburgh. Before he qualified he had another paper published, on the treatment of fractures of the wrist. He argued in favour of a new type of splint which he had seen used by Patrick Heron Watson (1832-1908) then an Edinburgh surgeon of considerable ability and drive. From this paper and others which appeared after he qualified, it seems that Tait and his fellow students were often given considerable clinical responsibility. It is also apparent that he kept meticulous records of all he saw and did as a student.

Not much can be gleaned of the background to his studies. His amusements may well have been restricted by his lack of money. He probably lived most of the time with his family. We know little of how he spent his vacations, but he probably worked part of the time in the hospitals. In the summer of 1863 he acted as an unqualified assistant to Dr. McFarlane of Drymen (Tait's father had come from Drymen). We know also from an entry in the Medical Directory that he held for a time the somewhat vague appointment of "Clinical Assistant, Ophthalmological Wards, Edinburgh". Although he had many acquaintances in his student years there is no evidence that he made any intimate friends; indeed, some of his fellows may have thought him an odd character and as medical students are apt to do, suspected his intense industry and enthusiasm. Amongst his student contemporaries was David Simpson, the promising elder son of Professor Simpson, who (the son) died prematurely in 1867. In 1890 Tait met up with Professor McLean of Michigan, but there are few references by Tait to any other fellow students.

Life as a medical student was hazardous. While working at the City Fever Hospital in 1861 Tait became seriously ill with a fever which was probably typhus. Although he recovered, three of his fellow students succumbed to this epidemic. In an address given in 1890 Tait recalled his experience of another typhus epidemic:[15]

> I was six months in Dr. Warburton Begbie's typhus ward at the top of the old Edinburgh Infirmary. I never stayed in that ward more than three quarters of an hour without coming away with a headache, and an hour's stay produced loss of appetite and vomiting.... but I got into the way of timing myself to half an hour and taking a long walk round Arthur's Seat every evening, so that I escaped the dire disease, whilst six of my colleagues took it and five of them died.

For the Edinburgh student there was a choice of medical societies offering a mixture of serious and social activity. The Royal Medical Society, the oldest in the British Isles, was founded in 1737.[16] Membership of this society gave considerable standing and it was unique in that it provided a forum for discussion between students and graduates. A presidency was regarded as the peak of a student's or a young graduate's career. In Tait's time David Simpson was one of the moving spirits and he became President in 1864. In the records of this society the name of Tait appears only once, participating in a discussion in 1866. He does not appear in any list of members and, perhaps because of his short spell as a matriculated university student, he was less likely to be elected. He was, however, from October 1863 until he qualified in 1866, an active participant in the smaller and less select Hunterian Society, one of many other contemporary societies.

The Hunterian Medical Society of Edinburgh was founded in 1824.[17] Its object was "the cultivation of Medicine and the Auxiliary Sciences:

and the business shall consist in reading and discussing Communications and Essays connected with these subjects. Instead of such papers, however, the Society may substitute a Debate on any of the subjects above indicated". This was not a very large society; fewer than twenty attended the meetings in Tait's time. From the Minute Book it seems to have been rather austere. There were fines for late arrival at meetings and for failure to present a paper on the advertised day. When a paper was offered and accepted a critic was appointed a week before the delivery, so the speaker could expect anything from praise to complete demolition of his views. All in all it was educational for the student. Medical topics were sometimes abandoned for debates with other societies; these were on such matters as the evils of nicotine or on capital punishment. There was an annual supper, but this seems to have been the only frivolity. Tait read four papers to the society, his subjects ranging from excision of the knee joint to eye diseases. There was a debate on the relative merits of acupressure and the ligature and Tait was in a minority when he spoke strongly in favour of Simpson's method. His chief, McKenzie Edwards, was one of the few seniors who participated in the meetings. In the 1865 to 1866 session Tait was elected President. The title of his inaugural address is not recorded in the Minutes, but Tait later recalled that it was on Darwin's theory of Evolution and that it brought him into unpleasant relations with the University authorities. Although it may have been less influential than the Royal Medical Society, the Hunterian Society provided Tait with experience in debate and argument, an experience which certainly bore fruit in his subsequent stormy career.

Scattered throughout Tait's subsequent lectures and papers there are numerous references to his early medical training, not always flattering. Twenty-seven years after he entered the medical school he recalled in an address at Birmingham:[18]

> My earliest surgical recollection is still very vivid. The operating theatre of the old infirmary was crowded, every seat even of the top gallery was occupied. There were probably seven or eight hundred spectators, for Syme was to operate on a gluteal aneurysm. He was then at the zenith of his fame, and in the very best of his powers, his hand as steady and his eye as true as it ever had been—incomparably the best surgeon I have ever seen. He entered the theatre with the recognised procession of assistants—house surgeons and dressers—and was greeted with a subdued murmur of applause. The spectators included men of all ages and ranks in the profession. Very many who

[*sic*] had come from great distances to see the great feat—like Bickersteth, of Liverpool, who came specially to assist, if I remember rightly—and, of course, there were many boys like myself from fifteen upwards. The patient was put to sleep, Syme buttoned up his dress-coat, turned up his sleeve, I saw a rush of blood, and in a few minutes the placing of the patient in the carrying chair and a round of applause announced the conclusion of the operation.

I have often wondered since and now I wonder more deeply why we gathered in such numbers to see that operation. The boys did so from curiosity and in ignorance. I am sure I did, and my ignorance was in no way lessened for I saw little of the operation, and I understood less. The older and more experienced spectators went mostly from curiosity and perhaps to be able to say that they had seen the great surgeon do this great deed. Some six or eight men were there, like Bickersteth, who might some day be called upon to operate for a gluteal aneurysm, and they were the only legitimate spectators. All the others had far better have been away.

In those days the first-year students were turned into the operating room and I believe this practice is still continued, to learn how operations are done before they know the names far less the relations, of the structures concerned. In the dissecting rooms our greatest feat was to display skilfully the fancifully named layers of fasciae which, if we had been really operating for hernia, we certainly would never have troubled about: or to remember the varieties of troublesome perineal arteries with which not one per cent of us would ever have any practical anxiety.

The strange thing was that this nonsense was encouraged by our teachers—nay it was carried into the examination hall. . . . the College of Surgeons was the great manufacturing agency for those practitioners of England and Wales who had the care of all the ailments of British humanity. . . . In order to receive a certificate which enabled the candidate to deal with scarlet fever and pneumonia, he had to answer questions about the internal iliac artery and how it might be tied.

Such criticisms had a sound basis and Tait amplified on these themes on other occasions. In his address on Surgery at the Annual Meeting of the British Medical Association in Birmingham in 1890 he castigated the teaching of the minutiae of anatomy to the student.[19]

I remember we had to learn that the dissection of the anterior cornu of the fourth ventricle of the brain which was backwards, outwards, downwards, forward and inwards and we were enabled in the most

> improper way to remember these important facts by the word 'bodfi'. Has 'bodfi' ever served any of you at the bedside? Is there any conceivable condition of human accident or ailment in which 'bodfi' could assist you to relieve your patient?. . . . Again let me remind you of the terrible task that we had to face in committing to memory the names and relation, the ligaments and points of contact of the bones of the wrist and of the ankle-joints. . . . I cannot imagine that the committal to memory of these peculiarities can in itself constitute any kind of mental training and I think the present system of anatomical training involves a gigantic waste of time and much frittering away of serious mental effort.

Such scorn of the frequent use of the mnemonic in the study of anatomy and of the excessive detail required of the student emphasises Tait's subsequent very practical approach to medical education. It is clear that even as a student he saw the defects of the curriculum. The day of the theatrical performance in the operating room is gone, but perhaps even Tait would think now that the anatomy course had been emasculated to an extent that students have too little knowledge of the human frame!

In retrospect Tait saw much to condemn but he completed his training at a time when movements to improve medical teaching had only begun and the overthrow of empiricism and the old philosophies had not been completely achieved. The teaching of physiology, for example, remained almost stationary at this time and was infiltrated with theological doctrines.[20] One current textbook of physiology opened with the simple statement: "Every organ of the body has a specific constitution and is regulated in its action by fixed laws appointed by Divine Wisdom". Tait must have been scornful of such influences, for as a student he was greatly intrigued by the theories promulgated by Charles Darwin. This influenced his philosophy and religious outlook. In this preoccupation he showed at an early age how he was stirred by the great scientific revolution of these years, while many of his contemporaries clung obstinately to the old doctrines.

When the time came, the final examinations offered no great problem, and Tait qualified L.R.C.S. and L.R.C.P. Edinburgh on May 11, 1866, aged almost exactly 21.[21] He was not eligible to take the University qualification of M.D.

Very likely recommended by Simpson in the summer of 1886, Tait went as an assistant to Dr. John Balfour Kirk (1826-1882) of Bathgate. Kirk had qualified M.D. of Edinburgh in 1847. He was well-known to

Simpson, who all his life maintained close contacts with Bathgate, his birthplace. Kirk had the reputation of being an exceptional doctor and had been in practice in Bathgate since 1850. In his obituary it is recorded that he was an able surgeon, a "fearless chloroformist" and one who had gained the respect and trust of all his patients despite the exertion of an iron discipline over them.[22] For a newly qualified doctor the attachment to Kirk's busy country practice was ideal and Tait stayed for a year absorbing all that Kirk could teach. In this short period Tait sent seven communications to the medical press. Three were on fractures of the wrist, augmenting the account he had already written as a student, and rather boldly suggesting that Abraham Colles' classic description of wrist fractures in 1814 was inaccurate and that the eponym "Colles' fracture", already widely accepted, was quite unjustified. Two further notes were on acupressure, in which he emphasised the value of this technique for the single-handed country practitioner. From such notes it is clear that he assisted Dr. Kirk at many operations and that he was already doing some surgery on his own. On one occasion he went to the scene of a railway accident and amputated a crushed leg at the knee joint, using acupressure to control the major vessels. He described how he had to take the victim back to his home and how he nursed the amputated stump on his knee to diminish the pain caused by the jolting of the carriage. The amputated stump healed rapidly and Tait considered this to be a triumph for acupressure. Unfortunately, the patient died two or three weeks later from a brain abscess (this might, in fact, have been caused by sepsis at the amputation site).

Undoubtedly here was a young man anxious to make his mark. He was not averse to some advertisement: a flow of articles, short notes and letters to the medical journals, which had now started, was to continue throughout his lifetime. His first entry in 1867 in the *Medical Directory* is illuminating, for it occupied as much space as that accorded to Professor Syme on the opposite page! It reads "L.R.C.P. and L.R.C.S. Ed. (Univ. Ed.). Pres. Hunt. Med. Soc. Edin". Then follow the titles of three of his early papers and the hint of more extensive authorship – "and various contributions to other journals". The entry for the next year records that he had become a member of the Surgical Society of Ireland. He visited Ireland briefly in the summer of 1867, saw the Dublin hospitals, met some of the Dublin surgeons, and learnt much that was new in this active school.

It seems likely that already a surgical career was his choice. He was near enough to Edinburgh to keep in touch with developments there, but whether or not he attempted at this stage to gain a footing in his own school is unknown. Surgical openings were limited and the competition was great. Any sponsorship by Simpson might not have been advantageous, for in 1867 Simpson was going through a difficult period during which he was under attack from many of his colleagues. Family influence and nepotism were of great significance as far as hospitals and university appointments were concerned, and Tait had no helpful connections. It is not surprising therefore that in the summer of 1867 Tait did what so many Scottish doctors have always done; he crossed the Border to take up a surgical post in Wakefield, Yorkshire.

CHAPTER II

Apprenticeship in Wakefield (1867-1870)

Lawson Tait was appointed house surgeon to the Clayton Hospital and Wakefield Dispensary in July 1867.[1] The hospital had only 12 beds but the dispensary provided a large outpatient practice.

In 1854 the Wakefield General Dispensary and the Wakefield Home of Recovery, both founded in the previous century, had combined to form one establishment endowed by Mr. Thomas Clayton, Mayor of Wakefield. He had purchased a house off the North Gate and other houses were soon acquired in Dispensary Square to provide increased accommodation. In 1875 the hospital moved to a new site. The original buildings are now demolished, but one house still stands adjacent to the site and may have been used by the hospital staff. The 18th century brickwork, the heavy tiles of Yorkshire stone and the oak beams reveal the style of the early hospital. Even for its time it must have been an inadequate and antiquated structure. From its foundation it received generous support from the local people.

Wakefield around 1870 was an expanding industrial town of 21,000 inhabitants, the centre of an agricultural community which provided wool for its main industry. It had the unenviable reputation of being one of the most unhealthy towns in the British Isles. In 1870 Dr. Radcliffe, Medical Officer to the Privy Council, reported on the shocking state of its sanitation, the appalling housing conditions, the indescribable pollution of its river, the Calder, and the dubious purity of its water supply.[3] In one of the crowded yards behind the main street Dr. Radcliffe found, in seven houses, 15 victims of enteric fever of whom two had already died. He acknowledged in his report the help he had received from the local doctors. One was Dr. James Chrichton Browne, medical officer of the local asylum, and the other was the house surgeon to the Clayton Hospital, Lawson Tait. When the report appeared there was an angry leader in the local paper. Admittedly the mortality rate in the town was little worse than that in similar towns in England, but certainly much of Radcliffe's report was justified.

It is not known why Tait chose to go to Wakefield, but his predecessor Dr. Fothergill had qualified a year or two before in Edinburgh. There were two honorary surgeons and two honorary physicians. The surgeons, Dr. Fowler and Dr. Walker, were both general practitioners and did not have specialist diplomas in surgery. Thomas Walker (1826-1918), although qualified M.R.C.S. Eng., had trained in Edinburgh. Tait was now most likely bent on a surgical career and soon, in the absence of any real competition, he took on the bulk of the operating. Later he recalled: "I had a mass of surgical material at my disposal and a kindly and indulgent staff, under whose direction I was permitted to make full use of it". This certainly is confirmed by the publications he presented in the next three years. No specialty was barred to him, and his medical and surgical activities had the widest range.

In 1867 surgery had reached a crucial phase. The introduction and acceptance of general anaesthesia had widened the surgeon's repertoire. This expansion had by no means been immediate, for there was a fear that in operating on the unconscious patient surgeons would expand their activities too rapidly and perhaps dangerously, that they would be tempted to achieve the near impossible, and that they might prolong operations unduly with great risk to the patient. Speed had been the hallmark of the successful operator in the pre-anaesthetic era. It had been a matter of pride to complete a major amputation in two or three minutes, and indeed there was still an unfortunate tendency to applaud such virtuosity. It was recorded of one surgeon that he "with one sweep of the knife cut off a limb as well as three fingers of his assistant and the coat tails of a spectator"!

The influence of general anaesthesia on ovariotomy (or removal of an ovarian cyst), the only accepted major abdominal operation in 1867, had at first been negligible. In the British Isles in the 10 years before the introduction of anaesthesia in 1846, more successful ovariotomies were achieved than in the subsequent decade. It is true there were other explanations for this rather surprising figure, but it does suggest that at first the benefits of anaesthesia were not reflected by a rapid advance in surgical endeavour.

Tait went to Wakefield well indoctrinated concerning chloroform, well trained in its administration, and aware that surgical procedures could be multiplied and expanded by its use. He had worked closely with Simpson and he had seen Syme and other Edinburgh surgeons accept the advantages of chloroform over ether. In England opinion varied as to the respective merits of ether and chloroform, but it could be said that surgeons there were equally divided, at times dogmatically or acrimoniously, in support of one or the other anaesthetic agent.

As far as general surgical technique was concerned Tait must have absorbed much of the basic teaching of Syme, whose textbooks were widely accepted in Scotland and not without influence in England. Tait would have observed Syme's insistence on cleanliness, unusual at the time, which if not very near the aseptic surgery of the future did allow a remarkable degree of success in what was a rather limited surgical repertoire. Tait was still imbued with Simpson's ideas concerning haemostasis and in 1867 was a strong advocate of acupressure.

Syme was undoubtedly conservative in his teaching. The preface to his *Observations in Clinical Surgery* reveals his cautious attitudes:[4]

> . . . . at no period in the history of surgery has there been so much occasion for information of this kind as at present, since the profusion of vague and verbose compilations, together with the mass of crude speculation and reckless misrepresentations with which the medical press has of late years teemed, have so bewildered the minds of most men as to render them incapable of discriminating between the good and evil of what they read. There hence results a painful feeling of uncertainty with constant straining after novelty as the wheel of fashion revolves, so that sound doctrines, instead of becoming firmly established through time, are apt to be relinquished and replaced by the silly suggestions of presumptuous folly.

Syme was certainly suspicious of novelty. He saw little merit in the use of the microscope. He would not accept the notion that pathology required special teaching, and he denied the necessity for a Chair of Pathology in Edinburgh. If he appeared over-cautious and antagonistic to change there was need for someone of his authority to criticise the surgical writings which were then appearing in great quantity, and which were too often of poor quality. There was a tendency to rush into print with new theories which were ill-founded or with operative results which were poorly documented or inadequately followed up. Too much attention was devoted to claims for priority and it was not unusual to find pages in the journals filled with rival texts set side by side to prove that one surgeon had plagiarised the other's writings.

In surgical history the year that Lawson Tait went to Wakefield was the most notable of the century. In 1867 Joseph Lister first published his discovery of an antiseptic system of surgery under the title "On a new method of treating compound fractures, abscesses etc.".[5] Before Lister's discovery, most surgeons had accepted with resignation or complacency the terrible morbidity and mortality which attended injuries or operations as the result of sepsis, evinced by the scourges of erysipelas, septicaemia, pyaemia and hospital gangrene. Although in 1847 Ignaz

Semmelweiss (1818-1865), and other obstetricians before him, had demonstrated quite clearly that puerperal infection could be greatly reduced by the simple precaution of the attendant washing his hands when he came to the lying-in ward from a septic case or from the autopsy room. But the lesson was not learnt by the surgeon. This was partly because puerperal sepsis was not at first equated with wound sepsis, but in general the surgeon was uncritical and accepted his disastrous results as inevitable. He denied the desirability or possibility of achieving healing of wounds by "first intention" without sepsis, and the expression "laudable pus" speaks for itself.

Before the publication of Lister's work, the ravages of infection were attributed to vague theoretical causes such as a miasma in the air. When Lister went to Glasgow as Professor of Surgery his interest in the etiology of surgical sepsis was stimulated by the challenge offered by the appalling conditions in the Glasgow Surgical Hospital where he had to work. The significant clue came to him when he heard, quite fortuitously, of the experiments of Louis Pasteur who (by 1864) convinced the scientific world that fermentation phenomena in wine, milk or other fluids were the consequence of inoculation with minute living organisms or germs which pervaded the atmosphere. Lister repeated Pasteur's experiments in a simple form and showed how urine in flasks would remain sterile indefinitely, provided the particulate matter in the outside air could not enter. He was well aware that a simple fracture did not become septic, but that a compound fracture with communication with the air invariably did so. With simple logic he argued that Pasteur's "germs" were the cause of putrefaction in wounds. His first object was to find a method of killing these germs. He could not use heat as Pasteur had done in his own experiments, but after numerous trials he chose the already known antiseptic carbolic acid. The first clinical experiments consisted of the application of undiluted carbolic acid to cleanse the wounds of compound fractures which were presumed to be already contaminated and to provide, by the application of impregnated dressings, a barrier against the admission of further germs. The technique was soon elaborated and improved with more dilute solutions or pastes of carbolic acid and finally with the addition of the antiseptic spray in an attempt to sterilise the air in the environment of the wound during operation or redressing. It was a natural corollary for the surgeon to wash his hands and his instruments in carbolic acid. The final achievement was to sterilise catgut ligatures in the same way. Lister's first published results in 1867, when he reported the astonishing figures of nine complete recoveries following his treatment of 11 compound fractures, established a principle which revolutionised surgical treatment. However, the general acceptance of his theory and technique was extremely slow.

Tait knew of Lister's work in Glasgow and must have read his momentous paper in 1867. He would have been aware also that Syme, in that same year, had written of the antiseptic system that it was "certainly the most important improvement in surgical practice of recent times".[6] Acknowledgement from one of such eminence so respected by Tait should have encouraged a critical and dispassionate look at Lister's work. However, there were personal issues involved. Although Tait had respect for Syme's opinions he was more readily influenced by Simpson, who saw in Lister's discovery little more than the advocacy of carbolic acid as an antiseptic in the management of wounds. Simpson went to great lengths to prove that Lister was in no way original in introducing this substance. Almost inexplicably, Simpson failed to grasp the principles which Lister taught or to appreciate the application of Pasteur's work. Simpson's attitude was certainly influenced by his personal quarrels with Syme and not least by Syme's vigorous opposition to acupressure which culminated in a dramatic occasion in his theatre. In front of the surgical class Syme tore up Simpson's pamphlet and consigned the remains to the basket reserved for surgical debris. All this had rubbed off on Tait and he inevitably, if weakly, was against Lister from the start. It is regrettable that two such able men were blinded by prejudice in this way.[7] For Simpson, who was near the end of his career, it mattered less. For Tait, however, this controversy had, as will be shown, considerable influence on his subsequent surgical practice as well as on his career. This is the subject of Chapter VI.

Tait's attitude to Lister's antiseptic method during his early years in Wakefield is indicated by a letter he wrote in 1868 in which he announced that he had given it up. He had at least given the method a trial, using it in the management of compound fractures. Twenty years later he recalled, perhaps with some exaggeration and some inaccuracy:[8]

> From 1867 till 1870 Lister had no more faithful disciple, no more devoted follower, than the unknown house surgeon at the Clayton Hospital. I spent my days with my hands soaked in carbolic oil, making carbolic putty and securing carbolic lac plaster. . . . Years after when I had fallen away from the faith the argument against me. . .was the assertion that I had never seen and never did understand Listerism. I had been to Glasgow to see it. I had carried it

> out more scrupulously than the master himself. I had suffered painful attacks of haematuria. . . . but with all my successes there occurred the old troubles, death from pyaemia, loss of cases which I could not understand if Lister's doctrines were true. I thought a royal road to surgical success had been opened to me yet I found myself floundering. . . . I began to fear that it was a science falsely so-called.

In a description of his experience in Wakefield of the treatment of abdominal abscesses, published some years later, Tait refers to his somewhat haphazard use of carbolic acid in these cases:[9]

> I may here observe that I was, at the time, an enthusiastic follower of the doctrines of Mr. Lister and as each new dressing came out I religiously applied it. In this poor man's case I poured in carbolic acid and oil, I rubbed it diligently through a mass of gangrenous tissue and nearly poisoned him.

When Tait became established in Wakefield he had had as good a grounding in surgery as could have been obtained in any British medical school. His rejection of Lister's work was admittedly unfortunate, but in a curious way the battle which he was to fight over this was a stimulus to his career. Certainly he was well equipped to evaluate or develop new ideas; he was not in the least likely to be orthodox, and most of all he was quite prepared to defy the opinions of the Surgical Establishment.

Tait rapidly widened his clinical experience and subjected it to careful analysis. He made himself well acquainted with contemporary opinions by wide reading, by attending the meetings of local and more distant medical societies and by discussion with his colleagues.

He wrote many papers during his three years in Wakefield. There was one on fractures of the femur, stimulated by a meeting with an American, Dr. George Smith of Brooklyn, who had much experience of such injuries in the American Civil War. From him Tait had learned of Buck's method of fixing fractures of the thigh by weight and pulley traction, with counter-traction provided by the weight of the patient on a sloping bed. Tait appreciated that this was a great advance on Liston's methods of fixed splintage which he had learned in Edinburgh. He made observations on head injuries, describing the eye changes due to thrombosis of the veins behind the orbit following trauma or sepsis.

The treatment of cleft palate and harelip was an early interest; by 1870 Tait had operated on nine children and developed his own ideas. He thought these congenital conditions were endemic in some districts of Yorkshire. He appreciated the importance of early operation in infancy to close the defect in the hard palate and so allow the infant to suck. He considered that speech problems were a secondary consideration. At first he operated without anaesthesia but then he found that he could use chloroform effectively for the very young infant. He had no hesitation in criticising the technique established by Sir William Fergusson, the accepted expert in this operation, and he evolved a method based on different principles.

Tait's epidemiological interests were demonstrated in a paper on the incidence of thyroid disease in pregnant women. He found that in the valley of the Calder thyroid enlargements were particularly common in women. Not a great deal was then known of the function of the thyroid gland but Tait at least realised its particular importance in the female. While some operations had been done before 1860 for the relief of pressure from large glands, there was not any real acceptance of the desirability of surgical removal of part or all of the gland. Tait limited his studies to the incidence of the condition, to observations on the histology of an enlarged gland obtained by autopsy and to a trial of the many ineffective medicines. He made no suggestion that operative treatment should be considered.

Following his short visit to Dublin he had become an enthusiast for the treatment of aneurysms by prolonged external pressure, a method popularised in Ireland by Reid but much criticised elsewhere. Tait described his own modifications of the technique.

In 1868 he wrote his last letter in support of acupressure and thereafter discarded the technique. In this letter, despite his work as a student, there is the first suggestion of an antipathy towards animal experiments. Hardly ever again did he use such methods, believing they had little relevance to human problems. He was to become an ardent opponent of vivisection.

About 1868 he made his first attempt to remove an ovarian cyst. By 1870 he had had at least three successes with this operation, but he was wary of publishing these achievements. Although in 1865 Spencer Wells had established this operation as a justifiable procedure, there was still a cautious approach on the part of many surgeons. Tait may have sensed that it might not redound to his credit if it became known that he, a very young man, had had the temerity to tackle what was still considered to be a dangerous operation. It was not until 1872 that he recorded nine cases, with only one death. He did this in a very brief and almost laconic letter to the *British Medical Journal,* giving no details of the cases. The total was small but his results must be seen against contemporary reports. The lowest mortality rates were 20 per cent in the hands of the Edinburgh surgeon Thomas Keith and 25 per cent in the hands of Spencer Wells.

Tait was to pioneer the surgery of gallbladder disease, and there is a report in Mayo Robson's monograph on gallstones, published in 1905, that Tait, when in Wakefield in 1869 "removed some gall-stones from a suppurating gall-bladder by slitting up a sinus discharging from the umbilicus." While this was not a direct exploration of a diseased gallbladder, the experience may well have stimulated Tait's later interest in this aspect of abdominal surgery.

Another experience had considerable influence on Tait's ideas about abdominal surgery. The full story of this was not published by him until 1890 in a paper entitled "The surgical treatment of typhlitis". The significance of this study in relation to Tait's contribution to the understanding of the surgical treatment of appendicitis is considered in Chapter V. In Wakefield he encountered several cases of acute abdominal abscess which, in retrospect, seem very clearly to have originated, in most instances, from acute appendicitis. At this time this clinical and pathological entity was scarcely recognised and Tait, like most other surgeons, diagnosed these abscesses as "caecal" in origin. He was indoctrinated in a disease known variously as typhlitis, perityphlitis or caecal phlegmon. In 1866, just before Tait went to Wakefield, there had been disastrous flooding of the town, to which event he attributed an outbreak of tubercular diseases of the lungs and the abdomen and, perhaps more correctly, a high incidence of typhoid. He operated on several cases of "caecal abscess" relating the condition in some to a previous attack of typhoid fever. Although he did a postmortem on at least one unoperated case, he did not at this time associate such abscesses with disease of the appendix. There had been sporadic reports of successful surgical drainage of abdominal abscesses but very few surgeons or pathologists suspected that these might originate from disease of the appendix. Tait was in advance of his contemporaries in that he had no hesitation in treating such abscesses by urgent drainage. Most other surgeons used non-operative treatment, often successfully, by poultices, purgatives or opium. From this group of patients Tait undoubtedly learned certain lessons which he applied later in the management of infective lesions of the female pelvic organs.

At this time absolute specialisation in gynaecology was unusual but the start of Tait's special interest in this branch of surgery is revealed by at least three papers. He wrote on the subject of the possible association of uterine disorders and epilepsy, a topic which for many years was argued vehemently amongst the gynaecologists. He described an autopsy on a patient who died after an operation (which Tait had performed) for strangulated hernia and he was intrigued to find that there was also a twisted ovarian cyst which he recognised as the cause of death. (It is rather surprising to learn that the relatives accepted an invitation to view the autopsy.) Most important of all was his description of the management of a case of the rare complication of complete inversion of the uterus, for this was read at a meeting of the Obstetrical Society of London on July 7, 1869. It was received with interest and discussed by such authorities as Tyler Smith and Braxton Hicks.

This was not the first of Tait's incursions to the London scene. While working at Bathgate, qualified only three months, he had attended a meeting of the Medical Society of London in October 1866 to hear a paper on the treatment of aneurysm by acupressure. It is recorded that in the discussion Mr. Tate *(sic)* gave strong support to acupressure and described the experimental work he had done for Simpson.[10] London was to see much of this dogmatic young man. At times he was to win respect but often he was to incur severe criticism and bitter opposition. He had been in Wakefield only three months when he presented a paper on the treatment of femoral aneurysm at the Leeds Medical Club. In all such activities he showed his determination to make his opinions heard, but there were probably many who regarded him as rather conceited and pushing for his age.

Some of these early papers showed a definite leaning towards a special interest in pathology. Tait tried to elucidate clinical problems by doing autopsies whenever the opportunity arose. When Professor Henderson retired in 1869 Tait was reported as a strong candidate for the Chair of Pathology in Edinburgh. This suggests that he was not forgotten in Edinburgh and that he was making a reputation outside of Wakefield. Later it was announced that he had withdrawn his candidature in favour of Bell Pettigrew (who became, in 1875, professor of medicine and anatomy at St. Andrews). Pettigrew was not appointed; the Chair went to William Sanders, a much more experienced pathologist than either Tait or Pettigrew. Tait's chances of gaining this post were not high, but if he had persisted in his application and been successful he would have inherited a situation of some difficulty. Henderson had embraced homoeopathy, which led to prolonged attempts to force him to resign from his Chair. Professor Syme and others in Edinburgh had done their best to abolish the Chair, believing that pathology was best taught by the surgeon and the physician. Simpson, on the other hand, appreciated the importance of specialised teaching in pathology and he may have persuaded Tait to apply. That Tait even considered applying for such a high post at the age of 24 shows that he was setting his sights high.

There were many other aspects of medicine in which he became interested. He wrote about chorea and, modelling his style on that of Simpson, preceded his account with a learned historical review. He described his experience in relieving intractable pain with the new drug chloral hydrate as an adjuvant of chloroform and morphine. He was involved in the study of a local outbreak of foot and mouth disease in domestic animals and he proved to his own satisfaction that, contrary to general opinion, if this exanthem attacked human beings it was not transmitted by contaminated milk. In such studies he had the help of his friend Mr. Naylor, the local veterinary surgeon.

Absorbed as he was in this busy and surgical practice, somehow he found time for other activities. It was a strong tradition amongst Victorian doctors that they should indulge in scientific or literary pursuits. Many made their names by their contributions to botany, zoology, geology and other such subjects. Not infrequently they attained the distinction of election as Fellows of the Royal Society by such research rather than by their medical activities. It was also in the Hunterian tradition that a doctor should expand medical science by the study of plants and animals.

In a less hurried world these doctors had more time on their hands, and perhaps their practices were less demanding than they are today. It may be significant also that the medical curriculum was less crowded and that the student had time to interest himself in topics beyond medicine. Many doctors were broadly educated, well versed in the classics, and often had taken an Arts degree before embarking on medical studies. There were few, in consequence, who did not participate in the activities of local societies devoted to natural history, archaeology and the like. Those who did have such interests were usually the leading lights of such societies.

Tait conformed to this picture while in Wakefield and later in Birmingham. His acute powers of observation and his insatiable curiosity thus found an additional outlet. Once more he showed an affinity with Simpson, who was an ardent naturalist from his boyhood and whose interests extended even to the problems of mining, engineering and sewage disposal! Simpson had a deep interest in archaeology and in medical history. He participated in the excavation of ancient burial mounds and of monastic ruins. He was an acknowledged authority on antiquarian matters and his general practitioner colleagues knew well that if he came into the country for a consultation he expected to view the local places of interest and that he would be ready to identify some curiosity turned up by the plough. It was said that when Simpson became a University professor his more learned colleagues on the Senate deplored his lack of a classical education and his unacademic background. It was suggested that he took up archaeology to prove that he was a man of culture! Tait, perhaps to impress his colleagues and his patients with his versatility, did likewise. He became a member of the International Congress of Prehistoric Archaeology and a Fellow of the Anthropological Society of London and published at least one paper on prehistoric remains in Scotland.

A letter to one of the medical journals reveals his preoccupation with Darwin's theory of evolution and demonstrates his detailed knowledge of the anatomy of the skulls of prehistoric man, a topic of considerable relevance to the understanding of the evolution of the human from the large apes.

A paper on evolutionary theory was published in 1869 in the *Dublin Quarterly Journal of Medicine.* This had the provocative title "Has the Law of Natural Selection by Survival of the Fittest failed in the Case of Man?". It was Tait's thesis that the advances of medical science favoured the survival of the unfit rather than the fit, so reversing the Darwinian theory as applied to animals. He wrote, "Medical science.... enables the diseased to live. Those whom it saves from dying prematurely it preserves, to propagate dismal and imperfect lives". There are other interesting asides which merit quotation and which emphasise that he was full of original ideas. For example, he has this to say about the maintenance of property and social position:[11]

> Of necessity the law of entail is now impractible. The success of the original maker of a family has put his immediate posterity beyond the necessity of entering the arena for the struggle for existence. . . .

> We shall find, and that I believe before long, that a system of life peerages, which must be introduced, will push the ancienne noblesse to the wall. . . .when those who, in the struggle for existence, have obtained the first rank in law, medicine, in all the arts and manufactures, will form one Upper House of Appeal.

His prophecy that the creation of hereditary peerages would be abolished has now been fulfilled. He was insistent, however, on the need for the protection of property and he expressed some of his philosophy in the sentence, "To whatever rank mankind may attain in development, it is essential that there should be individual inequality."

This paper shows his readiness to enter into argument, not unsuccessfully, concerning social and political questions. On the more specific subjects of heredity and evolution he later corresponded directly with Charles Darwin. His championing of Darwin's theory at times brought him into conflict with churchmen and with some of his colleagues.

Tait's participation in the social life of Wakefield is revealed in the columns of the local papers. He soon became active in societies such as the Mechanics Institute and the Church Institute. Two months after he arrived in Wakefield he gave a paper to the latter society and it went on for two hours! It was entitled "Britain in the Stone Age". This created a certain amount of scandal, for the Chairman had to chide the speaker for expressing opinions about the origins of men which were contrary to Old Testament teaching. Tait mollified his audience somewhat by stating that he did not doubt the existence of a Creator but he was merely suggesting that the timing indicated in the biblical account of the Creation was wrong. In the end he was complimented, rather grudgingly, on his learning and industry. There were other lectures which led to angry discussion. The *Wakefield Journal and Examiner* recorded in February 1868 that "Mr. Lawson Tait at last finished his voluminous lecture on Alcohol". It was voluminous for it went on for four hours. and Tait was rebuked for taking up so much time for a session which was allowed six hours, spread over two meetings at the Mechanics Institute. He expressed the view that crime and disease were not related to alcoholism, but that alcohol was a useful food. This statement brought on his head the wrath of the supporters of the Temperance movement, which was then at its peak. There was a long correspondence about this very unruly meeting and an anonymous contributor attacked Tait for his "mania for statistics" and for his refusal to argue with his opponents, whom he had described as the "paid teetotallers". Another critic commented that "The idea now and then came across my mind that I must be listening to some infallible prophet"; he thought that this dogmatic young man should abandon medicine and exercise his talents from the pulpit or in the law courts. Already Tait was incurring just the kind of criticism which was to be made in later years when he presented his ideas to the medical societies of London.

No one could give a paper at these societies without Tait intervening and often giving an opposite opinion. One unfortunate lecturer who spoke in lavish praise of Shakespeare's writings was told by Tait that most of Shakespeare's plays were written by another person and that the lecturer had exaggerated his importance. Tait, now a self-appointed literary critic announced "on psychological grounds I do not believe that Shakespeare could have written the absurd ghost scene in Hamlet and the play of Macbeth." (Presumably he approved of *Macbeth*). If he was opinionated and perhaps lacked respect for his elders, Tait certainly made an impact on this small community, and he could be depended upon to liven up any discussion.

In January 1868 Tait attended the Annual Charity Ball with Mr. and Mrs. Stewart and their daughter, whom Tait was later to marry. Mr. Stewart was a local solicitor, and it is clear from such accounts that Tait was involved in the social round.

Tait may have resided in the hospital, but it is more likely that he had lodgings in the town. It is possible that he lived with a Dr. Kemp, or at least very near to him. Kemp was a local practitioner who owned Westgate End House, where for at least 200 years doctors have, to this day, practised in Wakefield. The house still stands, an attractive building of mixed styles and undoubted antiquity in a secluded garden. Above the stables there is a large loft which Tait used as a dissecting room. It seems unlikely that anyone but a doctor would have allowed human dissection to be done on his premises, which supports the suggestion that Tait lived nearby. Many years after Tait left Wakefield, a local boy who later became a surgeon frequently took his friends up into this loft to terrify them with the grisly specimens and bones which Tait left behind. This loft was almost certainly the crude laboratory in which Tait did many anatomical and pathological studies during his sojourn in Wakefield.[12]

Despite his argumentative streak and his unorthodoxy, it seems that he got on well with his medical colleagues in Wakefield. He was called to consult with local practitioners in difficult cases, and he was apparently accepted as an equal by his seniors in the hospital. He developed a close friendship with Dr. Crichton Browne (1840-1938), the superintendent of the local asylum, which at this time was a more advanced mental institution than most. Crichton Browne (later Sir James Crichton Browne), had qualified in Edinburgh three years before Tait, and he became chief Visitor of Lunacy to the British Isles. He came of a family distinguished for its contributions to psychiatric medicine. He was the first to issue regular clinical reports from a mental hospital and he established in the West Riding Asylum near Wakefield the first research laboratory for nervous diseases. Tait must have found him to be a stimulating colleague and may well have collaborated in his research into mental conditions.[13]

After three years of intense activity in Wakefield Tait had built up a reputation as a surgeon of talent and original ideas. Clearly he could not be content with the position of a small town surgeon, unchallenged by others and without the stimulus of competition. He knew that to fulfil his ambitions he must move to a centre which offered wider opportunity. He was not uninterested in financial gain, for he was developing expensive tastes and was beginning to enjoy the luxuries of life.

To most rising young men London must have appeared to offer the best prospects of professional advance, but to Tait it may have seemed otherwise. He decided to go to Birmingham and it was said that he chose this city because it was in the centre of England. Perhaps he already had confidence enough to believe that he could dominate the surgical scene from a provincial city. Meanwhile, in June 1870 he gained the Fellowship of the Royal College of Surgeons of Edinburgh, thereby increasing his chances of achieving consultant status.[14] There is no indication that there was anyone of influence likely to further his cause in Birmingham. His establishment there in surgical practice was to depend on his own efforts, his supreme confidence, his capacity for hard work – and his ruthless determination.

CHAPTER III

Early Years in Birmingham (1870–1874)

In October 1870 Lawson Tait acquired the house and practice of Dr. Partridge situated on the outskirts of Birmingham. For a short time Tait was a general practitioner, but after two months he rented a consulting room in Waterloo Street and made it clear that he intended to establish himself as a specialist. The decision was a bold one, for he was unknown in the city. Most of all he needed a hospital appointment if he was to gain acceptance.

Birmingham had grown rapidly to a population of 380,000. It was a lively, thriving centre of industry and commerce, rivalling any other in the kingdom. Politically it was the home of the radicals and the free traders. There was a well-developed social conscience influenced by those such as George Dawson and the Chamberlains; there was also an active interest in the sciences and the arts. Already the city was a medical centre of some renown. For the eager young Tait the scene was very different from that of Wakefield and there were great opportunities to be grasped.[1]

A large general hospital and some smaller institutions had been established before 1800. Perhaps the most famous of Birmingham's early doctors was William Withering (1741-1799) who discovered the therapeutic properties of digitalis, derived from the foxglove. William Sands Cox (1802-1875) had, in 1825, established some systematic instruction for medical students, most of whom were apprenticed to local practitioners. Some sporadic clinical instruction had already been organised in the General Hospital.

In 1828 steps were taken, largely at the instigation of Sands Cox, to establish a School of Medicine and Surgery. The aim was to prepare candidates for the diplomas of the Royal Colleges and the Apothecaries Hall by exploiting the lavish clinical facilities which were available, without the necessity of students spending a year or more in London or Edinburgh. Not least it was stressed that "the distractions and allurements of the metropolis will not be thus prematurely presented to the young student". There was criticism in London, based on the notion that "certain young gentlemen" (Sands Cox in particular) were not established as private teachers and were too immature. Nevertheless the school was opened and in 1834 its status was enhanced by the grant by

William IV of the title of "Birmingham Royal School of Medicine". In 1843 the Queen's College of Birmingham was established by royal charter with faculties of Divinity, Medicine, Law and Engineering. In 1841 the Queen's Hospital had been founded, and this provided clinical teaching for the Queen's College students. Shortly after, a rival, the Sydenham College was created and linked for medical teaching with the General Hospital. This new college had the advantage that it was free from the rather excessive influence of the Theological Faculty, which was exerted in Queen's College and which had led to unfortunate bickering between the governing body and the hospital staff. Sydenham College prospered and the influence of Queen's receded until in 1868, by a happy compromise, the former was dissolved and the two main hospitals were combined under a Birmingham Clinical Board to organise all the hospital teaching required for a medical school.[2]

In 1870 there were two Professors of Surgery. Oliver Pemberton (1825-1897) had trained in Birmingham and then completed his medical education at St. Bartholomew's Hospital in London. He returned to his native city to become a surgeon to the General Hospital. He was much involved in teaching, being Professor of Anatomy from 1853 and of Surgery from 1867. Pemberton was a capable surgeon but after becoming coroner to the city he concentrated on medico-legal work. His few writings in surgery included "Clinical observations: the various Forms of Cancer", of which Sir James Paget wrote that it was "an example of surgery and good taste". Pemberton became a Fellow of the Royal College of Surgeons of Edinburgh in 1873 and was awarded the English Fellowship in 1878 as a Member of the College of 20 years standing. Thereafter he was a prominent provincial member of the College Council. When Tait came to Birmingham he found that Pemberton had considerable influence.

The second Professor of Surgery was Thomas Furneaux Jordan (1830-1911). He was the son of a Birmingham surgeon and trained in Queen's College. He became a Fellow of the English College in 1866 and was surgeon to the Queen's Hospital from that date. Although not physically robust he was an able operator who is best remembered for his method of amputation through the hip joint. He too was influential and served on the Council of the English College.

Of the older surgeons of repute Sands Cox had already left the scene. He had served the medical school well as a lecturer in anatomy and in surgery, but he quarrelled with his colleagues and retired from active practice in 1863. His ability was recognised by his election as a

Fellow of the College of Surgeons of England when in 1843 a large number of Fellows were created and most of the better known surgeons in the country were so honoured. In 1834 he had become a Fellow of the Royal Society. Although he had no contacts with Sands Cox, Tait must have been aware of Cox's role in establishing the Birmingham school.

Another notable surgeon, Samuel Langston Parker (1803-1871), was still in practice on the staff of the General Hospital when Tait arrived. Parker was held in considerable respect, although his contributions to surgery were not notable. He had held a Chair in Comparative Anatomy and was also a recognised authority for his writings on syphilis.

The Professors of Midwifery over this period were John Clay, Samuel Berry, and John Basset. Clay was well known (but not to be confused with Charles Clay of Manchester) for his interest in ovariotomy. for he had translated an important textbook on ovarian diseases written by the German gynaecologist Kiwisch, a work which had great influence in England. Samuel Berry was known to be an able and practical obstetrician who had much to do with the founding of the Women's Hospital which Tait was subsequently to make world famous.

These were men of some calibre, and there were other able surgeons and gynaecologists. It was no easy matter for a young unknown, having hopefully put up his plate. to break into consultant practice. It was not surprising, under such circumstances, that at first few patients came to Tait and that his finances were at a low ebb. In 1870 he applied, without success, for a consultant post at the General Hospital. Undeterred, he became active in supporting the establishment of a special hospital for women.

Throughout the country there was considerable opposition to the creation of special hospitals. In Birmingham the scheme was resisted by many of the consultants in the two large general hospitals. Despite all opposition, early in 1871 the founding committee purchased premises at 8, The Crescent, and vacancies for surgeons were advertised.[3] The influence of Tait in this campaign for a new hospital was probably not very significant, but by his support he at least made himself known to prominent citizens, such as Mr. Arthur Chamberlain, who were involved in this project. A rule was made that the surgeons appointed should hold the F.R.C.S. of England. In three months Tait prepared himself for this further examination which he passed in June 1871 just in time to get in his application, which was accepted. Two senior consultants, Berry and Furneaux Jordan, were elected, while Thomas Savage (1839-1907), Ross Jordan (? -1908) and Lawson Tait became junior surgeons.

Savage worked closely with Lawson Tait for many years, and when Tait became Professor of Gynaecology in Birmingham in 1887 Savage was elected Professor of Midwifery.

This rather makeshift hospital, the Birmingham and Midlands Hospital for Women, opened its doors to patients in December 1871 with only eight beds to be shared amongst this generous allocation of surgeons. In 1878 the hospital moved to Sparkhill and in 1905 it moved to its present location. Its subsequent expansion and reputation reflected the work done within it by Tait.

There was a parallel in London; Spencer Wells made his name in surgery by virtue of his attachment to one small Women's hospital, the Samaritan. The two hospitals were rivals, both contributing to the rapid expansion of gynaecology. It became a choice for those who aspired to work in this specialty as to whether they should attach themselves for training to the London or the Birmingham School.

If in some respects Tait's first (and only) hospital appointment in Birmingham had limitations, he made the most of his opportunity. For most of his life he was averse to operating in large hospitals, believing that surgery was much safer in a small institution. Nevertheless, a consultancy in one of the large teaching hospitals would have been advantageous, but this he never achieved.

Outside of Birmingham Tait, in 1873, was appointed consultant surgeon for the diseases of women to the West Bromwich Hospital. There were 24 beds and Furneaux Jordan, his senior, was the other consultant surgeon. Presumably Tait did some operating in West Bromwich and this attachment certainly increased his contacts with practitioners beyond Birmingham. For some years after 1874, he held the post of surgeon to the Skelton Private Asylum for Ladies; it seems unlikely that this offered him much in the way of surgical practice! In later life he was an Honorary Surgeon to the Brooklyn Hospital for Women, the Nottingham Samaritan Hospital for Women, the Wolverhampton Dispensary for Women, and the Women's Hospital in Liverpool.

Although Tait rapidly became recognised as a specialist, he continued to practise all branches of medicine and contributed increasingly to the medical journals. He wrote on many topics, such as tracheotomy in infants, the treatment of tuberculous abscesses in the neck by repeated tapping and the treatment of tetanus. There was an original note on the cure of inveterate eczema in a child by vaccination. In 1872 he published his first monograph, *On the Myoidema of Phthisis.* This was a short study of a curious muscular irritability observed in wasting diseases. Tait considered the sign had some diagnostic value and his book was quite favourably reviewed.

He became an active member of the now influential British Medical Association when he was in Wakefield. He attended assiduously the Birmingham meetings, taking a forceful part in debates, presenting papers and demonstrating innumerable specimens. At one meeting he showed the curious mixture of two breast tumours, the antler of a deer, and a peculiar lesion he had found in sticklebacks—such were his wide interests! He appeared at most of the annual meetings of the British Medical Association and was on the committee of the surgical section when this event came round to Birmingham in 1872. Such activity made him well-known locally; if this was a form of advertisement it was perfectly ethical and an accepted feature of professional life. There were, however, critics who came down heavily on any practitioner who overdid these things! In 1873 Tait arranged a conversazione on anaesthesia at his house, inviting reporters from the leading medical journals. The editor of the *British Medical Journal* expressed disapproval of this "offensive and invidious departure", and refused the invitation. Tait replied that at least he had not asked reporters from the lay press. This mollified the editor, but he indicated that Tait "had been warned".[4] There are hints that already he was building up some antagonism in London. The *British Medical Journal* had published a sequence of vituperative letters between Tait and two London surgeons, James Lane (a senior consultant in St. Mark's Hospital), and Arthur Norton (of St. Mary's Hospital). Tait had been called as a witness in a case over a charge of negligence brought against a dental surgeon and his evidence was quite contrary to that of his professional seniors. Perhaps rashly he criticised his colleagues in print, describing their statements as a "scandal to science". A terse reply followed:[5]

> We care little for the opinion of Lawson Tait and when that self-satisfied gentleman places himself on a high moral and scientific elevation and serenely sits in judgement on the conduct of two members of his own profession. . . .we feel compelled to question his title to the position he has assumed. . .

This small incident shows how, around 1870, the profession had not lost the habits of backbiting and slander in which it had indulged in earlier years, habits which often led to unsavoury litigation between doctors. It shows also that Tait could be rude and outspoken in his professional dealings. Such petulance did not endear him to London circles and some of the opposition which he was to meet when he presented his papers undoubtedly arose from personal antipathy towards him.

Tait was, however, eager to be accepted in London circles. While at Wakefield he had begun to attend meetings of the London societies and to mix with the leaders of the profession. In 1871 he was elected a Fellow of the Obstetrical Society and he read papers at this and the London Clinical Society. In 1874 he gave an account to the Medico-Chirurgical Society of his first successful operation for the removal of a large fibroid tumour of the uterus by the abdominal route. The chairman, Mr. Timothy Holmes, was rather critical of Tait having attempted such a dangerous procedure. However, Holmes was not well disposed to the younger man as he had crossed swords with him the previous year in an interminable debate about hospital infection. But this ebullient young man was beginning to make his mark outside of Birmingham and if some in London viewed him with suspicion a few were beginning to recognise his ability and originality.

He advanced rapidly in his career and his appointment to the Women's Hospital concentrated his interest on gynaecology. Recalling that he was still in his middle twenties, his contributions to this specialty at this time reveal a remarkable degree of boldness, originality and intensive research. He read the voluminous literature on his subject, not only from British and American sources, but also from the vast pathological and clinical records of German workers. At some stage he had mastered the German language sufficiently to translate and have published a *Compendium of Children's Diseases* by Johan Steiner. It is interesting to note that in his foreword to this volume, published in 1874, he announced that he had retained the centigrade scale used by Steiner for temperature records and had himself given up the Fahrenheit scale. It was to be about another hundred years before the rest of Britain followed suit!

Tait's boldness is illustrated in the way he now undertook operations which were the prerogative of relatively few experienced men like Spencer Wells of London and Keith of Edinburgh. He continued his work on ovarian cysts and began to perfect his own technique. His first success in the removal of a uterine fibroid has already been mentioned. In 1872 he reported his first abdominal operation to deal with an extra-uterine pregnancy, where an abnormally lodged gestation had survived to full term. He was not the first to do this operation, but when he presented the case to the Medico-Chirurgical Society Spencer Wells, on congratulating Tait, admitted that he himself had performed only three such operations.

Tait had no hesitation in applying himself to one of the most difficult problems, the repair of the disabling condition of rectal or bladder fistula, the most frequent sequel of crude obstetrical management. James Marion Sims (1813-1883), the American gynaecologist, had made a significant advance in this operation when he introduced the use of non-irritant metallic suture material about 1851, but the results in severe cases continued to be very discouraging. Tait employed a new suturing method, using the instruments he had evolved for cleft palate operations, and he had some remarkable successes. To cure this kind of case, often already subjected to many operations by other surgeons, was something which attracted favourable attention to a young consultant.

Tait's experience in the surgery of ovarian cysts demands more detailed comment, for the evolution of the operation of ovariotomy largely reflects surgical practice and concepts in the 19th century. The ultimate success achieved in ovariotomy opened the way to abdominal surgery of all other kinds. By 1872 Spencer Wells had done 500 such operations; he had toiled from 1857 to perfect his results and had fought a hard battle to establish the legitimacy of the operation. Tait's brief report in 1872 of a meagre nine cases has already been mentioned and may seem rather negligible in comparison with Spencer Wells' huge series, but there was still a very critical attitude to the performance of this type of surgery. Tait had left Edinburgh influenced by Syme who had, for most of his career, condemned the procedure. Syme himself had never attempted ovariotomy, and even in 1868, when he gave the annual British Medical Association address on surgery at Leamington, he was lukewarm in his support, despite the achievements of Thomas Keith and Spencer Wells.

Ovariotomy was first done successfully by Ephraim McDowell (1771-1830) of Kentucky in 1809.[6] His report was disbelieved in England when it was first published in 1817. John Lizars (1792-1860) of Edinburgh, who read McDowell's paper, in 1825 achieved one success out of four attempts. He was given little credit for this and the criticism he suffered for daring to perform such a hazardous operation deterred him from any further efforts. In 1841 Charles Clay (1801-1893) of Manchester did the first of a surprisingly successful series of ovariotomies, but he too failed to convince his colleagues, particularly those in London, that the operation was justified. A few other surgeons made sporadic attempts, some of which were successful. In 1850, at a debate in the Royal Medico-Chirurgical Society in London, there was a total denunciation of the operation. Not until 1857, when Spencer Wells did his first case, was there a revival. Gradually this determined surgeon achieved a degree of success which silenced the critics. His method involved the use of a crushing clamp which was applied to the severed pedicle of the cyst and which held the exteriorised stump on the abdominal wall. By this means Wells cut down the risk of peritoneal infection. This complication often developed with the earlier method of ligating the pedicle with a ligature (which was likely to be septic), returning the stump to the abdominal cavity, and bringing out long ends of the ligature to surface, as was the custom in amputations. The "long ligature" was hazardous in any operation, at the best causing a suppuration of the wound, and at the worst a fatal haemorrhage. In the pre-Listerian period Wells thus adopted a means of protecting his patients who underwent ovariotomy against the risk of peritonitis. In time, Lister's work, particularly with the introduction of the sterile ligature, made it safe to discard the clamp. Tait had much to do with this very important improvement in technique. From his experience of ovariotomy he went on to establish a variety of new abdominal procedures.

It is not quite clear exactly how Tait did his first ovariotomies. It is probable that he used the exteriorisation method, for originally he had considerable respect for Spencer Wells' opinions. However, in 1872, when Wells reported his fifth series of 100 ovariotomies to the Medico-Chirurgical Society Tait was in the audience and he showed some audacity in standing up to advise the acknowledged expert to discard the clamp and to use a technique now developed by Keith. The Edinburgh surgeon crushed the pedicle with an instrument known as an écraseur and then returned the stump, if all bleeding was controlled, to the abdominal cavity. Whether or not Wells, on this occasion, resented an unknown surgeon from the Midlands giving him advice is unknown. Soon, however, they were to become implacable enemies. Later, it will be recounted how Tait rapidly increased his experience of ovariotomy and how he achieved remarkable results.

While Tait's increasing experience of abdominal operations must predominate in an account of his early work in Birmingham he applied himself to many other problems in gynaecology. He published letters, notes, and articles on topics as diverse as intra-uterine therapeutics, the treatment of uterine inertia in prolonged labour and the relationship of epilepsy to menstrual disorders.

Of his early contributions to gynaecology the work which brought Tait the most publicity was an essay which he entered for the Hastings Prize given by the British Medical Association.[7] This was entitled "Diseases of the Ovary". It won him the award and at the Annual Meeting in London in 1874 Sir William Fergusson presented him with the Hastings medal. Fergusson made complimentary remarks on the quality of the essay and expressed the hope that the author would fulfil the great promise he had shown in his work. It was a long essay, printed in the *British Medical Journal* in five instalments. In it Tait reviewed the existing state of knowledge of the anatomy, physiology and pathology of the ovaries. There were some details of his own experience of operations, such as ovariotomy. It was not a very original paper but it must have cost him much labour. When eventually he published it as a small monograph it was well received.

As a background to all this surgical endeavour, there was in the seventies a continued and bitter controversy concerning the merits of the antiseptic system of surgery. Tait's participation in this battle is the subject of a separate chapter, and it is sufficient at this stage to refer only to his early utterances on the subject. At Wakefield he had tried Lister's techniques and found them wanting. He stated again in 1871 his opinion of the antiseptic method "that its merits have been overrated and its good results, which are quite as uncertain as those by other means, are due to the greater care of the cases and to the exclusion of the air".

Closely linked with the whole question of wound infection was the argument which raged concerning "hospitalism". Simpson had coined this term in his intensive study of the risks of surgery in large, crowded hospitals as compared with those in small hospitals or in the patient's home. Simpson's statistics were greatly criticised and regarded by some as inaccurate. His unfavourable conclusions regarding surgical practice in the large hospitals drew a storm of protest, for many believed that, if they saw these statistics, patients would be afraid to enter the hospitals. There was the additional concern that the rich patrons of charitable foundations would withdraw financial support. Shortly after Simpson's death Tait announced that the family had entrusted him with all Simpson's papers concerning hospital infection and that he intended to complete "his great master's work". By his continued support of Simpson's views Tait incurred the wrath of those such as Timothy Holmes, who deplored the "undigested heap of figures" on which Simpson had based his conclusions. Tait replied vigorously to Holmes' attacks, admitting a bias in favour of Simpson, but affirming that he had checked the statistics and found them to be accurate. Tait greatly resented that London surgeons should lay down the law about such matters and he castigated Holmes for his derogatory criticisms of the provincial and the country surgeon.

Behind all these arguments about "hospitalism" was the great question as to whether or not hospital mortality rates would be improved by the application of Lister's methods. Tait refused to accept this possibility. How much his judgement was coloured by resentment of anyone daring to take sides against Simpson is uncertain but it must be emphasised that Tait was not alone in his opposition to Lister. If, 100 years later, these vituperative confrontations may seem petty this controversy nonetheless dominated the surgical scene in Tait's time.

It is difficult to imagine how, with all his professional activities, Lawson Tait had much time for anything else. He soon became involved in medico-political affairs, whether local or national. He was always ready to express his opinions, which he did with great force. Medical education of women, for example, then a matter of much controversy, did not escape his attention. He spoke at length on this subject in Birmingham, and in general he was in favour of women becoming doctors; he thought that Birmingham "with its support of free trade should be liberal in its views". He was aware of Elizabeth Garret Anderson's abortive attempt to matriculate in the faculty of medicine in Edinburgh in 1863, despite sympathetic help from Simpson and other teachers, and of the long struggle in Edinburgh and London before women were admitted to medical schools in equality with men. He did have some reservations which would not be very acceptable in some quarters today for he stated categorically that the female brain was inferior! He quoted the somewhat dogmatic statements that "la femme est une malade", and that "a woman was incapacitated twenty per cent of the time". He considered that most women doctors would get married and that their expensive medical training would be wasted, an argument which perhaps still has some relevance. He concluded that the entry of women to the medical profession would always be small in proportion to that of men. But he was very fair and it is interesting to note that very soon the Women's Hospital had female house surgeons, and also that Tait himself for long employed a lady anaesthetist. He took the trouble to go to Zurich, where female medical students were accepted, and he described how there was not the least embarrassment because of their presence on those occasions when diseases peculiar to the male were demonstrated, in Tait's time indeed a delicate matter which exercised many of his colleagues!

Tait developed firm views, coloured by his studies of the theory of natural selection, concerning the education of women. In later years, he was to write:[8]

> . . . .I may own myself an advanced advocate of women's rights; at the same time I cannot help seeing the mischief women will do to themselves, and to the race generally, if they avail themselves too fully of these rights when conceded. It may be and probably is, a very gratifying circumstance for a young woman to go to a College, and show that she could take as high a degree as a man. . . . to fulfil the necessary conditions she will tax herself to such an extent as will, in all probability, make her functions imperfect. To continue the Career begun at College, she must deny herself the congenial occupations of a wife and the pleasures of maternity, and thus she robs the human race of what it wants most, brain-power on the part of the mother. To leave only the inferior women to perpetuate the species will do more to deteriorate the human race than all the individual victories at Girton will to benefit it. . . To hear an elderly maiden lady read a learned paper on mathematics may be a gratifying circumstance, but it is largely qualified by regrets when we speculate what superior children she might have produced if she had been a little less learned in books.

Tait was appointed lecturer in physiology and biology at the Midland Institute in Birmingham, where he taught a class of ladies the elements of these subjects. His frank expositions were criticised, not least his firm support of the Darwinian theory, regarded in many quarters as against the established religion and even as heretical.

Tait became friendly with George Dawson (1821-1876), a notable Baptist preacher who was responsible for the establishment of Free Libraries in Birmingham. Dawson was deeply involved in local politics and in social reform. He had founded the *Birmingham Morning News* in 1871, a paper which had considerable circulation with its strongly Liberal views. The friendship with Dawson may have established Tait's political attitudes but, more importantly, he was asked to contribute leaders and articles to Dawson's paper and so acquired an additional source of income when he was earning very little from his private practice.

In 1871 Tait married Sibyl Anne Stewart, to whom he had become engaged while in Wakefield.[9] She is described as a sweet, gentle lady who "through good and evil days devoted her life to promote his welfare and happiness". She took considerable interest in all his work and became adept as his proofreader. Tait's mother came to join what must have been an erratic household subservient to her dynamic, restless and impetuous son. To the long roll of doctors' wives who have tolerated the irregular hours, the disturbed social round and all the other disadvantages of sharing life with single-minded, often selfish, medical practitioners, perhaps particularly surgeons, the name of Mrs. Lawson Tait must be added in letters of gold. There were no children of the marriage, but there was understanding and true affection between them which persisted to the end, despite crises which might well have disrupted their alliance.

After four years of hard work and now only 30 years old, Lawson Tait was firmly established and recognised throughout the country as one who would make his mark. His most important contributions to surgery were to come in the next ten years. He burst like a meteor over the surgical scene. Like a meteor he was to burn out rapidly but in this transit light was thrown into dark corners and his influence was far-reaching.

CHAPTER IV

The Productive Years. Gynaecological Surgery (1875–1885)

Towards the end of 1873 Tait moved from Waterloo Street to Great Charles Street, purchasing a larger house in a more fashionable district. His practice was increasing, not only in Birmingham, but also throughout the Midlands. Both free and fee-paying patients were admitted to the Women's Hospital but it was more lucrative to consult and operate in the private houses of the rich. Tait was not averse to increasing his income but he always remained generous to the less affluent and accepted such fees as they could afford. He treated his hospital patients with solicitude and kindness.

The enormous expansion of Tait's surgical work from around 1874 is reflected in his writings and in his presentation in the next decade of an astonishing range of new ideas and procedures. Although he quickly began to occupy a dominating position in gynaecological circles – and did indeed regard himself as a specialist in this branch of surgery – many of the contributions he was to offer were in the wider field of general abdominal surgery. This was a field ripe for development largely because of the experience of the ovariotomists. It can be truly said that of all the lessons learnt by the ovariotomists most speedily and to the greatest effect. Spencer Wells, who in 1880 reported his thousandth ovariotomy
effect. Spencer Wells, who in 1880 reported his thousandth ovariotomy
was, in contrast, slow to expand his repertoire in the surgical attack on other abdominal conditions. He did do the first elective removal of the spleen in England in 1865 (the patient died eight days later) and he did have a share in pioneering other abdominal operations, but he failed to persuade others that such new procedures were valid and in some matters he remained very conservative.

That Tait, in this period (despite his concentration on gynaecology), was able to accumulate so much experience in general abdominal surgery is readily explained. It was not in his nature to confine himself to one branch of surgery to the exclusion of others. The modern fashion of extreme specialisation had not yet evolved, and indeed specialisation was frowned upon by most. Tait was unlikely to pass on to another surgeon any case which presented a challenge or a new opportunity, for he did have a fair conceit of himself! Inevitably he was sent patients with abdominal tumours thought to be of ovarian or uterine origin. In some instances he knew very well that the initial diagnosis was wrong and in others he himself might be in error, but with his skill and boldness he had no hesitation in dealing with the condition as he found it; a lesser man might have closed the abdomen without taking any positive action. It should be recalled that many of the "firsts" of abdominal operations were achieved when a confident diagnosis of ovarian cyst had been made but at operation a courageous surgeon dealt with something quite unexpected. As early as 1825 John Lizars of Edinburgh, from his experience of four abdominal explorations for ovarian cysts, had expressed the view that "operation should be resorted to more often for volvulus, intussusception, internal hernia, calculus and other obscure diseases of the abdominal and pelvic viscera." Lizars, perhaps because of the vicious attacks made upon him, was not prepared to risk his reputation by putting this logical idea into practice. Clay of Manchester, a bolder surgeon, at an operation for a suspected ovarian cyst in 1843, found a uterine tumour and removed the uterus (but the patient died). The first successful cholecystostomy, or drainage of the diseased gallbladder, was done in the United States by John Bobbs of Indiana. He had diagnosed a huge ovarian cyst, but the tumour was a greatly distended gallbladder. In 1885 Spencer Wells did his first successful splenectomy, having suspected that the huge mobile spleen was an ovarian cyst. Such sporadic adventures into new techniques did not receive general acceptance, and it was largely Tait who was to persuade others that abdominal surgery could and should be expanded.

Up to about 1885 Tait's major contributions to gynaecology were in the pathology, diagnosis and operative management of ovarian diseases, of extrauterine pregnancy (or ectopic gestation) and of myoma (or fibroid) of the uterus. There was also his insistence on the necessity of urgent operation for acute gynaecological conditions. There was his advocacy of "gastrotomy", or as it was later termed, "laparotomy", as a diagnostic weapon in uncertain chronic conditions. Tait preferred the simpler term "abdominal section" to the inaccurate word "laparotomy". He wrote numerous papers on many other gynaecological topics, some important and some perhaps trivial. These covered such diseases as puerperal endocarditis, perineal repair, inversion of the uterus and vesico-vaginal fistula.

Few surgeons or physicians of any distinction, and a great many of no distinction, in this time of medical and scientific advance, resisted the temptation of writing a monograph or a textbook. This was a means of advertisement, not only to impress colleagues, but also to enhance a reputation in teaching students. The output, as today, must have overrun the demand and many such works sank without a trace. Only a few survived in new editions, but the medical journals were generous in the space given to reviews of even the most trivial offerings. It was not surprising that Lawson Tait should enter the lists. In 1877 his first major textbook appeared, entitled "Diseases of Women". On the title page is printed, "Dedicated to Thomas Spencer Wells in admiration of the brilliant work by which the art of surgery has been enabled materially to prolong human life". In later years Tait regretted having made such a dedication; he accused Wells of having altered the wording of the printer's proof and rewriting it to his own satisfaction! The *Medical Times and Gazette* decided that the work was not scientific, that it was quite unsuitable for the student and that the opinions, if often original, were too dogmatic, too personal and made few concessions to other experts. The reviewer suggested that Tait diagnosed conditions by some mystical "tactus eruditis" which could not be transmitted to others. The *Lancet* was derogatory and dismissed the book as "scrappy". The *British and Foreign Medical and Chirurgical Review* thought it was poor and badly arranged, although the author's exceptional experience was recognised. It may well have been that among the London reviewers there were some who disapproved of Tait and thought him to be an upstart.

Looked at critically today, the work *is* rather poorly written and ill-arranged. It incorporates in the chapters on ovarian disease most of the author's earlier Hastings Essay, which had already been published. Nevertheless, there is much to interest the reader, not least the frank comments on subjects which were taboo to the Victorians. Tait comments on "the absurd social custom of the honeymoon". He suggests "it would be a great blessing to women about to be married if their mothers would give a little advice based on their own experience". He expresses his opinion that "the terrible carelessness of English women about the evacuation of the rectum is scarcely credible". In such comments he showed much understanding of women's problems, and in this sympathetic attitude there is once more a great resemblance to Simpson. In all his descriptions of the more distressing female complaints he appreciates the misery of his patients, the reluctance with which so many sought advice, the false modesty by which the doctor was so often prevented from asking necessary questions or making adequate examinations and the complete ignorance of female patients concerning their natural functions. There are pleas for sex education and for co-education, revealing how in so many ways Tait was so much in advance of his time. He expresses firm ideas about the upbringing of adolescent girls and attributes some of their disturbances to the deplorable custom of "keeping a young girl during her first efforts of sexual development seated upright on a music stool with her back unsupported, drumming vigorously at a piano". He insisted that in the crucial stage of puberty "for six months all instruction, especially in music, should cease".

The more technical aspects of gynaecology are dealt with very fully, recapitulating much of what he had already published in his numerous papers. As the reviewers commented the opinions are dogmatic and brook no argument. In his discussion on the major topic of the surgery of ovarian tumours he writes "To Mr. Spencer Wells must be accorded the credit of having placed ovariotomy in the position not only of an acknowledged operation but of one of the most successful of the great operations of surgery". It was not long before Tait recanted on this statement and accused Wells of having put back abdominal surgery by twenty years!

Although the work has many faults, it does not compare unfavourably with contemporary textbooks, and it was certainly more original. In some quarters it was well received, not least in America. If it did not enhance Taits's reputation greatly, nonetheless his humanity, his critical faculty, his wide experience and his complete disregard of established doctrine show clearly through the pages.

We have already recorded how, in Wakefield, Tait had begun to operate for ovarian cysts with success. His further experience was reported sporadically to the local societies in his early years in Birmingham. His technique initially followed that of Spencer Wells, with the use of the externally applied crushing clamp to meet the hazards of management of the ovarian pedicle. Soon Tait began to have doubts about this method and was veering towards intra-abdominal procedures for the crucial part of the operation. He tried the old-fashioned "long ligature", for which Clay continued for many years as the main advocate, but he (Tait) soon discarded it as dangerous. He tried a crushing instrument known as the écraseur (popularised in many operations by the French surgeon C. Chassaignac [1805-1879]), dropping the sealed-off stump into the abdominal cavity. However, his success with this method was mixed. When carbolised catgut was introduced by Lister in 1868 Tait tried it in one case: he cut the ends short and returned the pedicle to the abdomen. The patient died of peritonitis and Tait temporarily abandoned a principle which was soon to be accepted generally. In two cases he used silver wire to deal with the pedicle and he expressed some satisfaction with this method. He followed for a while the technique used by Thomas Keith of Edinburgh, whose results at this time excelled those of all other surgeons. Keith divided the pedicle, held it in a clamp, and patiently cauterised the cut surface by heat until all the blood vessels were sealed off, the clamp was removed, and the stump returned to the abdomen. Finally Tait adopted the method of simple ligation of the pedicle with clean silk or thread, with the ends cut short.

While Spencer Wells and most other ovariotomists at this time insisted that ovarian cysts should not be removed until severe symptoms and incapacitation had developed by pressure effects Tait now advocated their removal when first recognised, before the patient became a pathetic, emaciated invalid. There were many other problems which he clarified, such as the merits or demerits of tapping as a means of temporary relief (he was against this procedure), the use of drainage tubes, first advocated by Chassaignac and by Keith (this he favoured), and the choice of incision (he preferred a small incision, tapping the cyst if necessary to reduce its size before its extraction).

Unlike Spencer Wells, Tait did not record meticulously his successive hundreds of ovariotomies over the years, but he included such cases in his periodic reviews of all his abdominal operations. Some indication of the frequency and success with which he performed ovariotomy is revealed in one of his later papers presented at the British Medical Association meeting in Worcester in 1882. In this, he describes "One hundred consecutive cases of ovariotomy performed without Listerian details between November 1880 and May 1882". He had only three deaths in this series. This was a remarkable achievement, and a modern surgeon could improve only marginally on such results. In all his published series of ovariotomy (and of other abdominal operations), each case is readily identifiable and the name of the patient's doctor is recorded. As Tait wrote in one of his papers he provided "identification of patients in advance for critics who require it". Accusations were often made against Tait that he was dishonest in the publication of his results, but these can be discounted although his arithmetic was occasionally a little careless! Such was the suspicious and critical attitude of his time that if any doctor had seen his name linked with a case which was inaccurately reported he would very likely have publicised the fact.

In most of his reviews of ovariotomy from 1875 onwards, Tait attributed his success to the abandonment of Wells' method of exteriorisation by the clamp, to the adoption of Keith's method of cleansing the peritoneal cavity by irrigation (and, if necessary, the use of a drain), and to his own meticulous "hospital hygiene and discipline". It was perhaps unfortunate that in these accounts he was at pains to explain his success also by his complete rejection of Lister's principles (this matter is discussed more fully in Chapter VI). Tait's ultimate triumph is shown in a paper of 1886 when he recorded 139 ovariotomies without a death, an almost incredible sequence. All in all he must be credited with perfecting the technique of ovariotomy. He had, of course, advantages over his predecessors such as Clay, Spencer Wells and Keith, for they had to overcome an excessive prejudice against abdominal surgery of any kind; in addition, they operated on the more advanced and complicated cases, their anaesthetists were less skilled, their instruments and environment were cruder and when they pioneered the operation they had no conception of the origin of peritonitis or wound infection. Tait admittedly did take over an operation well on the way to general acceptance as a safe and legitimate procedure, but he was quick to tidy up the loose ends. Most of all, by his establishment of the simple method of ligating the pedicle, all the clumsy apparatus of the clamp, the écraseur, and the cautery could go on the scrap heap. The introduction of the simple intra-abdominal ligature had much to do with the introduction of safe surgery of other abdominal organs.

In his writings on ovariotomy Tait, rather unfortunately, could not resist an increasing urge to denigrate some of those who had pioneered the operation. In particular, Spencer Wells came under attack. Tait quite failed to appreciate that the clumsy method of exteriorisation of the pedicle with a clamp was, in the pre-Listerian period, much the safest technique to adopt, for it avoided returning the almost inevitably septic stump and ligature material to the abdominal cavity. When Spencer Wells had entered this field of surgery in 1857 he understood clearly the truth of a statement made by another pioneer, Baker Brown: "It's the peritonitis that beats us".

It has already been noted that Tait initially had a great respect for Spencer Wells and had acknowledged his considerable contribution to surgery. About 1873, the two surgeons were undoubtedly in a friendly relationship. An Australian visitor, Dr. Richard Tracy, records in his diary of that year that, when in London, he drove with Tait to Wells' elegant country house and estate at Golders Hill where he spent a congenial evening. Two weeks later, Tracy went to Birmingham with Spencer Wells. They lunched with Tait, and then the party went on to see Wells remove an undiagnosed abdominal tumour, which turned out to be a huge spleen. The spleen was removed but the patient died the next day. Soon, however, the friendship between these two great men deteriorated and they were never reconciled.[1]

With monotonous regularity the correspondence columns of the medical journals between 1875 and 1895 were filled with letters concerning the question as to whom priority should be given for the revival of ovariotomy after 1860 and its final acceptance as a safe operation. The editors had often to delete statements of extreme rudeness or those which might lead to litigation, but there remains in these letters a degree of vituperation almost unexcelled in any other medical controversy of the time. While belittling Spencer Wells' contribution Tait was always at pains to applaud the achievements of Clay of Manchester, who indeed was given little credit by anyone else in his lifetime. Between 1842 and 1857 Clay alone had persisted in attempts to improve and popularise ovariotomy. Tait also supported Keith of Edinburgh and acknowledged his very important work. Less convincing were Tait's recurrent efforts to credit Houston of Glasgow with a successful ovariotomy as early as 1701. Houston's case is simply not acceptable and Tait, it must be said, showed some nationalistic prejudice in attributing a "first" to Houston in Scotland rather than to McDowell in America!

The management of ovarian cysts had become a major preocuppation in the minds of surgeons and gynaecologists of the time and for a while there was remarkably little attention devoted to the possibility of dealing with all the other well-recognised pathological conditions of the ovaries and tubes by operation. Admittedly it was much easier to recognise a large simple cyst by clinical examination than to diagnose solid tumours or infective conditions with accuracy. Further, there was an attitude towards all operative interventions on the female reproductive organs which led to almost hysterical opposition. Even the surgeons who dealt with cysts were often stigmatised as "gelders" who, like veterinary surgeons, practised crude sterilising or spaying procedures. There was considerable moral objection to any operation which might conceivably alter the personality or the physical appearance of a woman. Most of all, the idea that the removal of functioning ovaries could ever be justified, met with extreme opposition. In consequence, large numbers of unfortunate women suspected of having painful and advanced ovarian or tubal disease were condemned to a ritual of useless and often painful treatment by applications of caustic materials, by cauterisations, by operations on the cervix, by a strange variety of electrical stimulations (perhaps occasionally of remarkable psychological benefit, but never curative), and by quite irrational general medication with toxic drugs. Such treatments sometimes produced debility or discomfort worse than that of the original disease.

Despite the fact that he had studied the pathology of ovarian diseases in considerable depth, Tait based some of his ideas on a gross misconception of female physiology. To the end of his days he persisted in a belief that the ovaries had nothing to do with the initiation of menstruation. He believed that in some mysterious way it was the tubes and not the ovaries which triggered the cycle of menstruation. His reasoning was somewhat nebulous:[2]

> All that I have said further in the shape of a tubular theory of menstruation is that the tubes are the starting point of the process. I never said that they were the cause. That they are the starting point is proved by the clinical fact that the characteristic symptom of tubal occlusion and distention is premenstrual pain.
>
> If the tubes are the starting point of the menstrual phenomena it is not unreasonable to suppose that their removal will be an effectual method of stopping it altogether. . . .
>
> . . . . I do not see how it is possible to advance any speculation as to the cause of menstruation other than it can exist in a nervous mechanism and there, for the present we must leave it.

He rather vaguely described a nerve which lay in close relation to the tubes and which controlled the uterine changes associated with the menstrual cycle. Time and again he made statements such as "the ovaries have little or nothing to do with menstruation and render it highly probable that the tubes are largely concerned. . . .". It seems possible that he had gained support for his argument by seeing cases where both ovaries had allegedly been removed completely and yet menstruation had persisted. He did not appreciate that if the smallest fragment of an ovary was left intact this would produce hormones which influenced uterine function. With an obstinate adherence to his tubal theory he rationalised the situation by advocating that if a tube was removed, then the ovary might as well come out also, because as far as conception was concerned, the remaining ovary was useless. As a corollary, if the ovaries were removed there was no point in retaining the tubes!

Before the end of the century, surgical excision of diseased ovaries, as well as those associated with gross cyst formation, became commonplace, to the great relief of many women. Lawson Tait was largely responsible for this radical change in attitude. There is some argument as to whether he was the first deliberately to remove a small diseased ovary diagnosed as the cause of severe pain. The priority does not greatly matter, although for years this was the subject of much argument. It is sufficient to credit him as an important pioneer in this new surgical approach. In 1871 Tait was asked to see a patient by Dr. Hall-Wright (a Birmingham doctor who later stimulated Tait to operate for ruptured ectopic gestation). This woman of 42 had suffered severe pelvic pain for years and when Tait examined her he found that the left ovary was slightly enlarged and extremely tender. In February 1872 he removed the ovary and cured the patient's symptoms completely. The pathological examination of the specimen suggested that this was a small chronic abscess of the ovary. In retrospect, this may not seem to have been a very epoch-making operation, but at the time Tait knew that the condition was unlikely to prove fatal but that his reputation would suffer greatly if anything untoward had happened as a result of the operative intervention. He did not report this case until 1879 and when in later years the controversy concerning priority raged around him, there were some who alleged that he had not made this undoubted break-through in gynaecology. However, if he had made this delayed report dishonestly, as was averred, his assistants, whose names appear in the record, would very likely have joined in these accusations. Tait certainly stated often that this early success led to his interest in the surgical management of inflammatory diseases of the ovary and tubes, an interest which resulted in some of his most significant contributions to gynaecological practice.

Before Tait did this operation, there had been chance examples of surgical removal of the ovaries for conditions other than large cysts. James Blundell (1790-1877), of Guy's Hospital, a thoughtful contributor to the solution of many surgical problems, in 1825 tried to persuade his colleagues that exploration of the abdominal cavity need not (as was then thought) cause fatal peritonitis, and he forecast that the removal of normal or diseased ovaries would readily be accomplished. There existed, from ancient classical writings and from the studies of anthropologists, a vast literature on the subject of male and female castration. In primitive tribes such as the aboriginals of Australia, removal of the ovaries was practised for ritual reasons. The subject greatly intrigued the gynaecologists of the Victorian period and it was discussed at great length. What was originally a topic of historical interest and of philosophical curiosity in earlier years became, however, in later years something immoral and lewd to be quoted against those surgeons who had the temerity to practice ovariectomy on their patients.

It is confusing to try and sort out the nomenclature applied to the ovarian operations which Tait and his contemporaries introduced. First of all, the word "ovariotomy", suggested originally by Simpson to Clay to describe the removal of an ovarian cyst, is inaccurate as it implies cutting into the ovary. In the 19th century, however, "ovariotomy" meant one thing only—and that was removal of a cyst. In practice sometimes the cyst alone was removed, as it was separate from the ovary; more often the ovary was involved by the cyst and so the ovary was removed also. In time the purists of language described removal of the ovary as oophorectomy or ovariectomy according to whether the ovary was normal or diseased. Tait strove to solve the confusion by referring to excision of the uterine appendages, for he usually removed both tube and ovary whatever the reason for the operation, sometimes on one side only and sometimes on both. Just to make things more complicated, these procedures were often referred to eponymously as Battey's, Hegar's, or Tait's operation. Such varied descriptions make it extremely difficult to evaluate or even understand some of the early writings on the surgery of the female pelvic organs.

After his early experience of the surgery of cysts Tait became involved in three other ovarian operations. First, he practised removal of functioning (and often normal) ovaries, either as a means of influencing obscure and often hypothetical conditions such as uterine epilepsy, or to control painful menstrual disorders, or to influence the growth or symptoms of uterine tumours. He, or any other surgeon who undertook this type of operation was immediately open to severe criticism or censure, since the removal of the functioning ovary was seen as a crude and indefensible spaying of the female. Second, Tait diagnosed a variety of solid tumours and localised inflammations of the ovaries which had scarcely ever been treated by radical surgery until he had the confidence to do so. Third, recognising in his practice in Birmingham a large number of women with large swellings involving both tube and ovary in an inflammatory tumour, often with abscess formation, he did what was quite unprecedented and excised these adherent and septic conditions completely by the abdominal route.

In 1872 Robert Battey (1829-1895) of Georgia, U.S.A., introduced a procedure to be known as "Battey's operation".[3] The normal ovaries were removed with the hope of curing certain neuroses or menstrual disturbances. As one medical historian states, "an evil practice was started innocently. . . . It was not Battey's employment of these principles but the over-enthusiastic application of them by his followers that caused the operation to fall somewhat into disrepute". The original indications for this operation were somewhat vaguely stated by Battey, but in particular it was advocated for insanity or epilepsy believed to be caused by uterine or ovarian disease. Battey stressed that in such cases the operation should be a last resort. But he was on dangerous ground in suggesting that such diseases did have such an origin. From early mythology and from the classical writers a strong belief had been inherited to the effect that conditions ranging from simple hysteria to insanity were related to the uterus (the word "hysteria" is derived from the same Greek root as is "uterus"). To any observer the alterations of moods of women in relation to the menstrual cycle could very understandably suggest that more advanced mental changes or nervous phenomena had the same origin. Isaac Baker Brown (1812-1873) had fallen into the trap of attributing epilepsy and insanity to some sort of trigger mechanism from the female organs and had become obsessed with the idea that such conditions could be cured by the removal of the clitoris, a minor appendage of the genitalia. When he published a monograph on the subject in 1866 he was blackballed by the London Obstetrical Society and viciously attacked by his colleagues. His practice was ruined and he died insane, forgotten by all. It could be expected equally that any proposal to remove the normal ovaries in similar circumstances would bring down the same bitter and damaging attacks on the heads of any surgeons involved.

Lawson Tait was cautious in applying this particular indication for removal of the ovaries, but he did for a while consider that there was a place for the operation. He reported a few successful results for what he termed "menstrual epileptic mania". In some of these cases he found pathological changes which were unexpected, as for example, "exanthematic cirrhosis of the ovary", and so he was able to stress that these were not true examples of Battey's much criticised procedure. But it was not easy to answer the frequent accusations that he had spayed his patients, and when he published some apparently successful results of ovariectomy for "menstrual epileptic mania", he was rated "the foremost advocate of spaying in women". It is all too clear that for a few years Battey's operation was done too often and with little justification and that if a patient died at the hands of a surgeon less capable than Tait the criticism was harsh and litigation was likely.

Battey put forward a rather better case in advocating removal of the ovaries for intractable and severe menstrual pain. By 1880 Tait had followed his lead, and in a series of 25 "oophorectomies" about a third were done for such indications. It is a little difficult to assess from Tait's reports just how successful and how justifiable these operations were.

There was another reason for removal of the normal ovaries. It had long been known that uterine fibroids, which could cause debilitating or even fatal haemorrhage, occasionally underwent spontaneous shrinkage at the menopause, with cessation of bleeding. It was reasoned that removal of the functioning ovaries might be justified to induce an artificial menopause. At the time a more direct attack on uterine tumours, either by local excision or removal of the uterus, was fraught with technical problems. Eventually, Tait and others mastered these problems and treatment by ovarian extirpation was discarded. As usual there was bitter argument about priorities. Tait alleged that he first did this operation on May 22, 1873, but that in five subsequent cases he was discouraged by the high mortality. However, he did the operation again in later years. Between 1879 and 1882 he performed it on 26 patients with two deaths and for a while he was convinced of its value. With his tubal theory of menstruation Tait always removed both tubes and both ovaries, while Hegar of Freiburg, whose name is usually given to the operation, removed the ovaries alone. Although Hegar was most likely the pioneer of this operation, Tait's experience was equally extensive and influenced British gynaecologists in particular.

After 1872, when he had removed a small inflamed ovary for the first time, Tait went on to accumulate a large number of cases where he had diagnosed either localised inflammatory lesions of the ovary or conditions of the tube, such as hydrosalpinx or pyosalpinx. More important, he began to advocate laparotomy or, as he preferred it, exploratory abdominal section for obscure clinical conditions. By his courage he was able to relieve many women of troublesome symptoms and chronic ill health who otherwise would have gone on indefinitely with the inadequate and often painful medical or electrical therapies of his more conservative colleagues. All such cases he published either in short notes or in his consecutive series of abdominal operations.

While his published experience and his frequent papers at the medical societies concerning the topics so far discussed always aroused interest and often much criticism perhaps his venture into the surgical management of gross inflammations of the uterine appendages led to more argument and disbelief than all the others. It had long been recognised that, as a consequence of infection originating in unskilled midwifery many women developed intractable inflammations of the tubes and adjacent ovaries, often with abscess formation. The condition resulted in chronic ill health, in sterility and in painful and trying symptoms. Occasionally, the fortuitous development of an acute abscess which was managed by surgical drainage might lend relief, but most victims of these conditions were condemned to years of useless medical treatment, and for those who were forced to pay for the privilege of private care, financial disaster. Similar conditions were not uncommonly a sequel of gonorrhoeal infection for which, at that time, there was no specific treatment. The chronic complications of this venereal infection, which was rife in all classes, simply could not be prevented. Tait encountered a very large number of such distressing cases in his hospital and private practice in Birmingham. Although the London gynaecologists knew of these different chronic conditions, for some reason they did not seem to diagnose them very often nor to recognise that conservative management was useless. Tait repeatedly gave papers and demonstrations in London in an attempt to indoctrinate his colleagues in his beliefs, only to be rewarded on one occasion by Spencer Wells' remark that "he never saw such cases, perhaps they all went to Birmingham". Some such patients *did* indeed go to Birmingham from London, simply because they were dissatisfied with their treatment and were aware that in Tait they would find a surgeon who had the reputation of doing something positive to help them. When this happened Tait unfortunately was too ready to publish the case and emphasise the manner in which some London surgeon had mismanaged it. As he was not averse to publishing the name of the surgeon he was often fortunate to escape litigation!

On one occasion Tait published the details of a patient sent to him from abroad and who had a long history of illness associated with chronic uterine or ovarian disease. Tait diagnosed a gross enlargement of the ovaries and tubes, which he associated with chronic infection, and he advised operative treatment. The patient asked if she might consult Spencer Wells. With some effrontery and perhaps undisguised glee Tait published Spencer Wells' report:[4]

> I can detect no organic disease of her uterus or ovaries. . . . it is very doubtful how far removal of her ovaries would affect the state of her nervous system, supposing she recovered from the operation of removal. I think more good might be done by change of air and mode of life, and some German baths and mountain air, than by surgical operation.

The lady did not accept this advice and came back to Lawson Tait for help. The latter found, as he had forecast, a gross pyosalpinx or abscess of the tube, removed it and cured the patient. Tait may not have been the only surgeon of the time to expose his colleagues' misjudgments or errors, but he did rather overdo this kind of thing, and his ungentlemanly behaviour hardly enhanced his reputation. On the whole Spencer Wells took these attacks with remarkable coolness, often ignoring them completely. His strongest weapon was his studied neglect in all his writings and speeches of any mention of Tait's numerous positive contributions to surgery or to gynaecology.

Technically, it was one thing to remove a large ovarian cyst or to excise a healthy ovary and tube, but it was quite another thing to attempt to eradicate the adherent inflammatory mass arising from chronic infection of the appendages. Tait undoubtedly developed an expertise and technical skill which few of his contemporaries possessed. He had a sense of touch which allowed him to separate tissues without causing serious bleeding or damage to vital structures. It was no easy matter to free these diseased tissues, and the surprising thing is that he used a very small incision for this operation.

In one of his numerous descriptions Tait writes:[5]

> I had very soon found that no kind of light helped me in the least and that my eyes were practically of no use to me at all in these operations. . . . I had to put my eyes at the tips of the index and middle finger of my left hand and now the whole of my operations—and very ghastly proceedings are constantly being encountered amongst them—are performed through an incision not more than two inches long.

Despite all difficulties the operation was done with speed, a necessity more pressing in Tait's time than today with modern anaesthetic techniques. All who worked with Tait commented upon his dexterity in this procedure. Unfortunately, his individual skill was not so easily transmitted to others, and it is possible that some of those who were tempted to embark on the surgery of this particular condition found themselves in real trouble.

In 1882 a paper entitled "Diagnosis and treatment of chronic inflammation of the ovary" first publicised Tait's ideas about the surgical management of this neglected group of cases. The title was not entirely apt, because he was really discussing advanced inflammatory conditions of varying origin whereby the tube and ovary were converted into a chronic adherent and painful mass. He began this paper with an attack on the useless therapies which were in vogue. Such treatments were almost entirely directed to the uterus with the employment of caustic applications to the cervix, medicinal pessaries, cervical dilatation, instillations of toxic or cauterising fluids into the uterus or surgical incisions into the cervix by the hysterotome. All were useless and, said Tait, the time had come to deal with the primary condition of the appendages by excision, especially as the relative safety of abdominal exploration had now been established. He was cautious, for he was prepared to give a reasonable trial to orthodox treatments. He insisted, however, "after a persistent trial of them without benefit there remains for consideration the removal of the diseased organs – a proceeding which is based on the soundest and most accepted rules of surgery." This, as always, was his text.

It took a long time for Tait to convince others of his views. In 1881 he showed to an astonished and rather incredulous audience at the Pathological Society of London a series of specimens from his first 19 cases, in which all the patients had recovered. He showed more specimens to the Obstetrical Society in 1882. At first there was frank disapproval, and once more (quite unjustifiably, as the ovaries in such cases must usually have been functionless) he was accused of wholesale spaying of his patients. He had to stress time and again that he knew perfectly well that he was not operating for a condition which would kill the patient, but that the time had come for surgeons to accept the idea that they must be bold enough to tackle diseases which produced chronic invalidism and intolerable symptoms.

The opposition was eventually worn down. This took some time, but after his repeated demonstrations of specimens to the Societies few could deny that "Tait's operation", as it was now known, was a remarkable advance. On one occasion he travelled to London with as many as 60 operative specimens; Alban Doran, working in the pathology museum in the College of Surgeons, was astonished to find specimen after specimen arriving there for exhibition.

Today, as it happens, these advanced inflammatory conditions of the uterine appendages are comparatively rare because septic complications after obstetrical procedures are largely prevented or eradicated effectively, and the advanced complications of gonorrhoea are now less common. This does not detract from the fact that Tait, by his determined efforts, proved conclusively to his contemporaries that they should abandon their pessimistic attitude to what was, in their time, a common cause of human suffering and that they should be bold enough to deal with such conditions by radical surgery.

Long before the 19th century there was an awareness and some understanding of the phenomenon of the development of a fertilised ovum in a site other than the uterus. The most common ectopic gestation was recognised to be in the Fallopian tube. Such a misplaced embryo could, but only rarely, survive, resulting in an abdominal pregnancy which usually terminated in the death of the child. More often a tubal pregnancy would rupture in the first three months and either give rise to a local haematoma of the tube and adjacent structures—a chronic condition—or would cause torrential bleeding into the abdominal cavity which, if untreated, resulted in certain death.

The chronic condition was not easy to diagnose. Tait became interested in this, studied it fully and gave his conclusions in a paper to the Obstetrical Society of London in 1873. In the same year he described to the Royal Medical and Chirurgical Society his first successful "gastrotomy" for an extra extrauterine pregnancy. He had removed a ten-month foetus by abdominal section; the child, of course, had not survived. Such an operation raised serious problems of bleeding if the abnormally placed placenta was detached. Tait solved this difficulty by leaving the placenta to separate spontaneously. In a discussion of this paper Spencer Wells said he would have removed the foetus by the vaginal route. This was the accepted method, but it had proved to be a difficult and dangerous procedure. Many surgeons did not operate at all for this condition; they preferred medical treatment, or they applied the electric current to "absorb the haematoma". Between 1878 and 1880 Tait removed advanced ectopic gestations by the abdominal approach in five instances, with only one death, and began to convince others that this was the best method of management. He clarified both the pathology and treatment of this chronic condition in numerous reports.

But it was in the management of acute haemorrhage from early rupture of a tubal pregnancy that Tait made one of his most notable contributions to surgery. Howard Kelly, writing in 1912, states that "the most dramatic operation in the whole realm of surgery is that for a ruptured extrauterine pregnancy, which lingered so long as one of the most hopeless and distressing ailments. Conquest of this malady was one of the most brilliant achievements of the last century". It is a little surprising that no surgeon before Tait was courageous enough to operate to try to control the acute bleeding caused by rupture of a tube.

The pathology was reasonably well understood, and it was all too clear that the patient died from acute blood loss, just as a patient would die from a severed major limb artery if no attempt was made at control. Many had at least discussed the idea of operation, but none had the courage of his conviction. In 1863 the problem was aired at the London Obstetrical Society when the account of a fatal case was presented. Spencer Wells was present and stated that "if it was certain that a patient was dying from internal haemorrhage owing to rupture of the sac of a tubal pregnancy he could see no sort of difficulty in the way of a surgical operation. . . . [It] would be simple: what the result would be was another question." In his textbook of 1877 Tait made some reference to this subject. He did not then think that the diagnosis of intraperitoneal bleeding from a ruptured tube was easy and he believed that "even if recognised in time, the operation for relief is as likely to do harm as good". He stated more explicitly that "if the case be one of tubal pregnancy, the doubt of a favourable issue to the operation for the arrest of haemorrhage. . . .is so great as to place it out of the question."

John Parry of Philadelphia published a book "Extra-uterine pregnancy" in 1876 and put the case forcibly:[6]

> A bleeding vessel, through which the red stream of life is rushing away, can be ligatured. . . . an aneurysm that places life in constant jeopardy can often be cured by proximal or distal ligature. . . . but here is an accident that may happen to any wife in the most useful period of her existence, which good authorities have said is never cured. . . . From the middle of the eleventh century when Albucasis described the first known case of extra-uterine pregnancy, men have doubtless watched the life ebb rapidly from the pale victim of the accident as the torrent of blood is poured into the abdominal cavity but have never raised a hand to help her. Surely this is an anomaly and it has no parallel in the history of human injuries. The fact seems incredible, for if one life is saved by active interference it may be triumphantly pointed to as the first and only instance of the kind on record. . . . The only remedy that can be proposed to rescue a woman under the unfortunate circumstances is. . . . to open the abdomen, tie the bleeding vessels or to remove the sac entirely.

Parry's book came into Tait's hands and may well have caused him to review his ideas about the possibilities of surgery in this acute catastrophe. It was, however, his colleagues in general practice who stimulated him to attempt the operation.

In the summer of 1881 Tait was called by Dr. Hall-Wright of Birmingham to see a patient who was thought to be bleeding from a ruptured tubal gestation. Tait agreed with the diagnosis:[7]

> This gentleman [Dr. Hallwright] made the bold suggestion that I should open the abdomen and remove the ruptured tube. The suggestion staggered me and I am ashamed to say that I did not receive it favourably. I saw the patient again. . . . again I declined to act upon Mr. Hall-Wright's request, [and] a further haemorrhage killed the patient. A post mortem revealed the perfect accuracy of the diagnosis. I carefully inspected this specimen which was removed and I found [that] if I had tied the broad ligament and removed the ruptured tube I should have completely arrested the haemorrhage, and I now believe that had I done this the patient's life would have been saved.

The lesson was learned, but it was not until January 17, 1883 that Tait saw another such case. Dr. Henry Shackman of Wolverhampton made the correct diagnosis and Tait reported:[8]

> The patient was clearly dying of haemorrhage and I at once advised abdominal section. . . . I wasted much time in trying to stop this haemorrhage, so that by the time the operation was finished the patient was practically dead. We got her to bed alive, and that is all that can be said. I thought much about the case, for it was a bitter disappointment: I thought I should achieve a triumph and I had only a failure. But my conclusion was speedily arrived at, that I had blundered—that the true method of operating in such a case was to separate adhesions rapidly, regardless of bleeding, and make at once for the source of the haemorrhage. . . . .

A second lesson had been learnt and digested. Lesser men might have hesitated to make another attempt, but on March 3, 1883 Dr. Edward Page of Solihull called Tait to a similar case and the patient was saved by urgent operation.

By June 1884 Tait had operated five times for such acute haemorrhages and only the first case had died. By 1888 he had saved the lives of 39 women and had lost only two. Without the benefits of blood transfusion this is a remarkable record. Tait gave his views on the pathology and treatment of extrauterine pregnancy to the obstetrical section of the British Medical Association at the Annual Meeting in Belfast in 1884. From that time onwards his opinions could scarcely be refuted. In 1888 he published a monograph entitled "Lectures on Ectopic Pregnancy and Pelvic Haematocele", in which he reviewed the subject very fully and gave complete accounts of his early cases.

The common condition of fibroid tumour of the uterus had been recognised for many years before 1870. This was seldom a killing disease, although in some cases the size of the tumour caused great discomfort and at times there was troublesome bleeding. The chronic nature of the condition and its occasional tendency to regress after the menopause combined to make the surgeon reluctant to undertake an operation for its relief. Lizars, Clay and other ovariotomists had occasionally found this condition when they explored the abdomen and some had dared to remove the uterine tumour. Such fortuitous operations usually involved a local removal of the tumour, which was relatively easy if it had a narrow stalk or pedicle. In some cases a partial removal of the uterus to include the tumour was done, but this was fraught with danger as there was no unanimity as to how bleeding should be controlled from the resultant raw surface of the remnant of the uterus. The idea of removal of fibroid tumours by hysterectomy (leaving the cervical part intact) was not generally acceptable, as there were unsolved problems as to how the cervical stump should be managed. Hysterectomy had been done in earlier years, for example by Kimball and by Burnham in America in 1853, but these were sporadic attempts at the operation. In 1863 Koeberle of Strasbourg did two elective hysterectomies for fibroid tumours, using a wire snare to control bleeding from the exteriorised cervical stump.

In 1874, when Lawson Tait (as recorded in the preceding chapter) presented his first successful operation for removal of a large fibroid tumour of the uterus by the abdominal approach, his contemporaries were lukewarm about the justification for such an operation and it was still generally regarded as excessively dangerous. Accordingly, many surgeons, including Tait, were at first glad to adopt Hegar's solution, by which he attempted to influence the condition indirectly by removal of the ovaries. Tait continued for some years to do Hegar's operation for fibroids. His gradual conversion to a direct operation for fibroids by hysterectomy was influenced largely by the work of Thomas Keith. In 1883 Keith published a series of 25 hysterectomies for fibroid tumours with only two deaths.[9] This mortality of eight per cent was very much better than that of any other operator at the time. Spencer Wells, for example, had recorded a 50 per cent mortality. It is curious that although Tait had so vehemently condemned Spencer Wells' exteriorisation operation for ovarian cysts Tait continued for some years to use a crushing clamp to control bleeding from the exteriorised cervical clamp in subtotal hysterectomy. This paradox is all the more strange because it was usually much easier to apply a clamp safely to an ovarian pedicle than to the uterine stump. Initially he used Koeberle's wire snare or serre-noeud, but he was not satisfied with his results.

Amongst other gynaecological procedures which Tait perfected rather than innovated in this fruitful period was that for repair of the perineum, and he was recognised as an expert in this operation. The technical details which he employed need not concern us, but he did evolve a method based on simple plastic principles, and his exceptional results depended not only on his consummate skill, but also on his careful after-treatment. This was an operation which he could demonstrate readily to his pupils and many came to him to learn his technique.

Appropriately, during this period of intense activity Tait brought out new editions of "The pathology and treatment of Diseases of the Ovary". These were expansions of his Hastings essay and they incorporated many of his more recent papers and case reports. The critics were now rather more generous, but there were still allusions to his excessive dogmatism. One reviewer wrote, "We doubt if there be any surgeon of the present day less trammelled by authority or bolder in risking his reputation than Mr. Lawson Tait of Birmingham".

There was reluctance to accord Tait due recognition for his achievements in the gynaecological field, and even those additional advances which he made concurrently in general abdominal surgery (reported in the next chapter) did not command the respect which, in retrospect, may seem to have been his due. Perhaps this was an inevitable reflection on his brash technique of presenting his views, his obstinacy, his insistence that he was always right, as well as his habit of attacking his colleagues. But there may have been also a strong element of jealousy, particularly in the minds of the London surgeons, who had begun to recognise that Tait was gaining a national and international reputation, not infrequently at their expense.

CHAPTER V
The Productive Years: General Surgery (1875-1885)

If Lawson Tait, in this the most fertile period of his career, had done nothing more than has been recounted in the previous chapter he would still have deserved a notable place in surgical history. Although his primary interest was in gynaecology it was inevitable that with his advocacy of the frequent use of abdominal exploration in his extensive practice he should widen his repertoire in surgery. So it was that in the decade between 1875 and 1885 he presented to the surgical world many new ideas by which he influenced the evolution of abdominal surgery, an evolution which was greatly accelerated in the last part of the century.

Up to about 1875, despite the advances in technique made possible by the use of general anaesthesia and by Lister's discoveries, most of the diseases of the digestive organs, the biliary system and the renal system, although often well understood in terms of pathology and symptomology, still remained from the therapeutic aspect in the realm of the physician. Few abdominal procedures were undertaken with real confidence, with the exception of operation for ovarian cysts. The common types of chronic external herniae were occasionally dealt with surgically although it was more usual to prescribe a truss than to do an elective repair. The acute complications of herniae were treated with some success but there was still a strong tendency to delay operation and to hope that opium, fomentations and the administration of enemata, of astonishing variety, would control such crises. If the contents of a strangulated hernia were grossly damaged and a length of intestine required removal the techniques were crude and often ineffective. Acute appendicitis, although it must have been frequent, was ill-understood. There were sporadic successful abdominal explorations for intestinal obstructions of various kinds, for adhesions, internal herniae and the like, but very often these cases were managed without need for operation and, if progressive, were invariably fatal. Of other acute conditions perforations of gastric or duodenal ulcers were well recognised but an attitude towards such situations had been expressed as early as 1843 by Crisp who wrote, "in the present state of abdominal surgery the operation of cutting into the abdomen and tying the aperture may be considered too quixotic to mention." This pessimistic view persisted for many years for it was not until 1891 that a surgeon was courageous enough to operate for perforated ulcer. The obstructive conditions of the colon were occasionally managed by making a colostomy. Penetrating wounds of the abdomen were sometimes treated boldly, particularly by military surgeons, but for every success there was a multitude of failures.

There was no established technique of elective surgery for such common conditions as malignancy of the stomach or of the bowel, for gallstones or for kidney diseases, although diagnosis was often remarkably astute despite the lack of X-rays and other modern techniques. There was an active interest in the management of bladder stones, a condition more common in the nineteenth century than it is now. The surgeon inherited a long tradition of dealing with such stones by a variety of approaches through the perineum, often with disastrous results except in the hands of a few highly expert lithotomists.

It is interesting to speculate what would have happened if Lawson Tait, instead of being appointed to a hospital for women, had had the opportunity of working in a general hospital where he would have cared for patients with a much wider variety of abdominal diseases. It is conceivable that in such circumstances his energy, his courage and his surgical expertise would have brought a revolution and advanced abdominal surgery much more rapidly than was the case. As it was, even with his relatively restricted practice, his contribution was considerable and W. J. Mayo had some justification in stating "the cavities of the body were a sealed book until the father of modern abdominal surgery, Lawson Tait, carried the sense of sight into the abdomen."

It has been told how Tait showed his contemporaries how many conditions of the female pelvic organs were best dealt with by the direct abdominal approach. His operation for advanced extra-uterine pregnancy is one example; his insistence that the useless medical treatments for chronic inflammation of the uterine appendages should be abandoned is another. His success with urgent operation for ruptured ectopic gestation was the culmination of his advocacy of a positive and urgent approach to all acute abdominal conditions.

Tait's influence on the development of the surgery of the biliary tract was of much significance. Gallstones and their complications had long been known and the subject of innumerable treatises by early writers. As early as 1743 Jean Petit, from his observation of three cases in which abscesses resulting from gallbladder disease were drained, advocated a planned operation to drain the gallbladder and so to deal with stones. John Bobbs drained a diseased gallbladder in 1867 and described how, on discovering that it was greatly enlarged, "the lower margin was cut through, when a perfectly limpid fluid escaped, propelling with considerable force, several solid bodies about the size of ordinary rifle bullets." He sutured the edges of the opened gallbladder to the abdominal wound and the patient recovered.[1] Kocher, in 1878, did a successful two-stage operation, packing gauze around the inflamed gallbladder and, when adhesions had formed, draining it four days later. Marion Sims did an elective operation to deal with a patient with obstructive jaundice and a rapidly increasing gallbladder enlargement (possibly due to malignant obstruction) in 1878.[2] He completed the operation by Bobbs' method but the patient died. Sims coined the word "cholecystotomy" for this operation.

In 1879 Tait was consulted about a woman who had developed a large painful swelling in the right side of the abdomen. There was some uncertainty as to the diagnosis, but a "dropsy of the gall-bladder" was considered. He opened the abdomen and recognised the enlarged gallbladder, emptied it with a needle and then removed a large gallstone through a small incision. There was another stone impacted at the cystic duct. This was impossible to remove by simple manipulation:[3]

> I thereupon performed a very careful and protracted lithotrity, chipping little fragments off the stone regularly all over its exposed surface till I had the satisfaction of lifting out its nucleus, I then passed the blade of a fine pair of forceps on each side of it, and by a gentle squeeze broke up the remainder and was then enabled to lift it out.... I washed the cavity out repeatedly, and took every precaution I could to be sure that no fragments were left. I then stitched the wound in the gall-bladder to the upper end of the abdominal wall.... and closed the rest of the abdominal opening in the usual way.

The operation was a success. No other surgeon at this time, if he had encountered such a situation, would have done more than drain the gallbladder. Tait was, however, adept at solving an unexpected problem such as was presented by the impacted stone. He reported the case to the Medico-Chirurgical Society in November 1879, realising its great importance. He thought it was the first successful operation of its kind. He had not read Bobbs' paper but he had almost certainly seen Sims' report, for he described the operation as a cholecystotomy. The discussion following Tait's account was lively. Mr. John Hulke (1830-1895), congratulated the speaker and drew attention to Petit's early paper. Spencer Wells said that he would prefer to apply a caustic to the skin over the swelling and wait for the stones to extrude spontaneously! In general there was reluctance to admit that Tait had once more presented something original and important. He quoted Marion Sims, "we shall make an early exploratory incision, ascertain the true nature of the disease and then carry out the surgical treatment that the necessities of the case may demand."

This was certainly the first operation of this type in Great Britain. In 1884 Tait recorded 13 similar operations, all successful. By 1892 he listed 71 cholecystotomies with only four post-operative deaths. In 1884 he had introduced a further suggestion; he had operated for obstructive jaundice and relieved the condition by crushing a soft stone in the main bile duct, without opening the duct. (Knowsley Thornton, in 1889 was one of the first to remove a stone by opening the duct). Langenbach of Berlin performed cholecystostomy (or removal of the whole gallbladder) for stones in 1882, but Lawson Tait did not approve of this advance which eventually was to replace the simpler operation of cholecystostomy.

While Bobbs may be given the credit of being the first to do a planned cholecystostomy, it was Tait who had much to do with convincing others that they should use this as a routine procedure, thereby paving the way for the rapid expansion of surgery of the biliary tract.

It must be conceded that Tait was somewhat obstinate and irrational in his ideas about future developments of the surgery of the biliary tract. He did not think removal of the gallbladder was necessary for the treatment of gallstones, for he believed that stones would not form again in a gallbladder which had once been drained. In this, or course, he was wrong. In extenuation it must be said that the type of case he dealt with was usually that of the patient with a very large swelling known as mucocele of the gallbladder, a condition which can be managed easily by simple drainage. He had limited experience of the management of acute jaundice and believed that most stones in the main duct passed into the intestine spontaneously and that the real problem arose, as in his first case, from stones in the narrow cystic duct. He did go rather far when he said "a surgeon might as well remove the urinary bladder to stop urinary stones," but he was apt to make his points by exaggerated statements.

Discussion soon began concerning other ways of dealing with gallstones. Spencer Wells suggested that the gallbladder should be opened, the stones extracted and then the gallbladder sutured. Tait very rightly disapproved strongly of this idea but he asserted, rather rashly, "The entire possibilities of the treatment of gall-stones and distended bladder are exhausted in Dr. Marion Sims' paper and no further extension of it is necessary." It is one of the curious paradoxes of Tait's career that having made such a positive step forward, as he undeniably did by establishing the operation of cholecystostomy, he then called a halt. There are other examples of such conservatism on his part – for example, his categorical denial of the possibility that chest surgery would ever progress beyond the simple operation of drainage of an empyema. Thus he states, "I cannot imagine any man in his senses would attempt to remove a human lung with a tumour in it. . . . for phthisis – removal of the lung would be a still more absurd proposal." In this discussion he did remark, with some justification, "I do not think the severest critic can say of me that I have any tendency to obstruct surgical progress." These prophesies about the surgery of the lung were, or course, quite wrong, but it has been rather a habit of distinguished surgeons, from Erichsen to Moynihan, to announce that surgery has reached its practical limits![4]

In his lifetime Tait did not receive much credit for his work on gallbladder surgery, but if his British contemporaries did not recognise his influence Ochsner in America wrote, "To Tait, more than any other surgeon of this period, is due the credit of placing the surgery of the liver and the gall-bladder on a firm basis."

Tait's huge practice inevitably brought to his notice some more unusual conditions. He encountered amongst these certain liver cysts the exact pathology of which must remain in some doubt. He described them variously as "hydatids" or "simple cysts". His biographer McKay suggests that these were true hyatid cysts due to the echinococcus, rare in Britain now but perhaps more frequent in the 19th century. Up to 1880 any attempts to operate for liver diseases were limited to the simple drainage of cysts or abscesses. In 1872 Langenbeck was probably the first to drain a suspected hydatid cyst.

In 1880 Tait was asked by Dr. Pike of Malvern to see a patient with a long history of illness accompanied by obscure symptoms and progressive enlargement of the liver. The diagnosis of hydatid disease was made by needle aspiration. Despite the emaciated and breathless condition of the patient on account of her huge liver Tait, with his assistant Mr. Raffles Harmer, agreed to operate:[5]

> Acting on the principle that I have already advocated. . . . of opening the abdomen in all cases where life was threatened, I had no hesitation in proposing abdominal section. . . . I opened the peritoneum and exposed healthy liver tissue. . . . Into this I passed a large-sized aspirator needle and evacuated a few teaspoonfuls of clear serum. . . . Removing the needle I passed a knife into its track. . . I enlarged the incision, this I did to the extent of three inches and the moment I freed my finger myriads of transparent globes of all sizes, from a pea to an orange, shot out, covering the table and the floor. . . When the tension was relieved I dug them out with a large silver gravy spoon, an instrument suggested to me by Dr. Pike, and this process took much more time than all the rest of the operation, and during its performance Mr. Harmer most carefully prevented any cyst entering the peritoneal cavity. . . . Finally I perceived that my gravy spoon was causing some haemorrhage from the inside of the cavity and I had to leave a considerable quantity of cysts. . . . The quantity of hydatid cysts evacuated is estimated by Dr. Pike to be about two gallons, and I think the amount is not exaggerated.

There was some troublesome bleeding from the cut surface of the liver but Tait controlled this, draining the area with a glass tube and suturing the edges of the opening in the liver to the abdominal wall. The patient made a remarkable recovery. She discharged more cysts through the drainage tube and then healed up. Two years later she was well and had married.

McKay, a surgeon practising in Australia where hydatid cysts are common, criticises some details of this operation but regards it as the first practical procedure for hydatid cyst. A similar operation, however, had been carried out by Lindemann in 1871 but Tait was probably unaware of this. Tait therefore deserves credit for independently devising a technique of 'marsupialisation' of a hydatid cyst so as to ensure continued and adequate drainage. The life cycle of the echinococcus was described by Knabbe in 1866, but Tait does not indicate that he understood the natural history of the disease. However, he seems to have appreciated the danger of releasing live cysts into the abdominal cavity, for he described how his assistant acted to prevent this complication.

When he reported this case at a meeting of the Royal Medico-Chirurgical Society at least one member of the audience said that it was a "triumph for surgery" and even Spencer Wells acknowledged that Tait's operation was much better than simple tapping, which was the orthodox treatment. Tait described what he had done as "hepatotomy". In a year he published four similar operations of which two, including the Malvern case, were undoubtedly for hydatid cysts, and two probably for simple developmental cysts. All four patients recovered. The series was small but important, for it showed surgeons that it was possible to deal effectively with such chronic diseases of the liver by abdominal exploration.

Tait's part in the evolution of the surgery of acute appendicitis is rather curious. There is evidence that he diagnosed this condition and operated successfully by removing an inflamed appendix in 1880. He did not publish the details of this case until 10 years later and, in consequence, he has not usually been given the credit of having pioneered this the most frequent of all operations for acute abdominal disease.

In the early part of the century there had been some clear expositions of the pathology of acute appendicitis, for example, by Burne of the Westminster Hospital and Bright and Addison of Guy's Hospital. Only a few surgeons, however, appreciated that right-sided abdominal abscesses were often due to appendicitis. A complete understanding of the pathology and presentation of acute appendicitis was confused because of the insistence on the part of some influential surgeons and pathologists, including the great Dupuytren of Paris, that acute inflammation in the right side of the abdomen arose from disease of the caecum and not from the appendix. While for years operative interventions for the consequences of acute appendicitis were confined to drainage of localised abscesses, as early as 1827 Melier of France had suggested that it might be possible to diagnose and remove the inflamed appendix before it burst to cause septic complications.[6]

It has been recorded in most accounts of the history of acute appendicitis that Mikulicz in 1884 was the first to suggest that the acutely inflamed appendix should be removed and that another German surgeon–Kronlein, in the same year–attempted this operation, but the patient died two days later. In his paper, Mikulicz acknowledged that Lawson Tait had stimulated his interest in acute abdominal surgery. The British surgeon Symonds did an elective operation for recurrent appendicitis in 1885 and Morton in 1887 was the first in the United States to diagnose and operate for acute appendicitis. However, in his paper (published in 1890), Lawson Tait makes it clear that he diagnosed appendicitis as early as 1880 and that he removed the acutely diseased appendix with survival of the patient. The paper was entitled "Surgical

Treatment of Typhlitis" and we have already referred to it in relation to Tait's experience in Wakefield of the treatment of acute abdominal abscesses. For some obscure reason he did not like the "new-fangled" term "appendicitis". He reviewed 24 cases of so-called "typhlitis", he defined this condition as "inflammation in the region of the caecum", attributing it in some cases to obscure lesions of the caecum, in others to typhoid infection and in the remainder to inflammation of the appendix. He considered that these three varieties of inflammation which caused acute right-sided pain could not be differentiated except by operation and stated:[7]

> . . . the conclusion is inevitable that the earlier operative intervention is employed the better for the patient. . . the risk of an unnecessary incision is so slight and the risk of a delayed incision so enormous that I am disposed to lay down the imperative rule that as soon as a diagnosis of typhlitis is established no attempt should be made by delay to ascertain which variety it belongs to but that a surgical operation in search of pus should at once be done."

Substitute "appendicitis" for "typhlitis" in this statement and Tait's advice holds as firmly today as when he wrote it. British surgeons were slow to accept such opinions; even at the turn of the century when Edward VII, just prior to the planned date of his coronation, was seized with appendicitis, Sir Frederic Treves and his associates, including the aged Lord Lister, temporised for several days. The royal appendix finally perforated and by good fortune produced a localised abscess which was eventually drained successfully.

Tait's account of his historic case deserves reproduction:[8]

> A.D. 17 . . . began to have ill defined pain in the right groin in May 1880 . . . . in August it became very much worse and when admitted to hospital in September 1880, there was peculiar crackling to be felt by the fingers over the swelling . . . the whole of the abdomen was swollen and the child lay with her knees drawn up so that I was under the impression that there was a general peritonitis from rupture of the caecum or vermiform appendix. I opened the abdomen in the middle line to explore and ascertain if there was anything wrong in the peritoneum but there was not. I then made an incision over the caecum and opened a large abscess extending deeply down towards the brim of the pelvis, and lying bare in the cavity was the vermiform appendix. It was black and discoloured and gangrenous.

> I therefore snipped it off, and inverted the stump into the cavity, stitching the inverted peritoneal surfaces together with fine silk, then fastened a drainage tube deep into the pelvis and closed the wound.

The girl recovered from what was clearly an advanced condition with a well localised abscess following perforation of the appendix. The "crackling" which Tait was astute enough to detect was likely due to gas in the abscess. In such advanced cases it is seldom possible to locate the diseased appendix and to remove it completely; indeed, it is usually safer not to attempt to do so. Rarely, as in this case, the appendix is found and can be removed. Perhaps Tait was rather lucky to get away with the operation he performed. He included acute appendicitis in his differential diagnosis, he operated urgently and he removed a gangrenous appendix. This is the first recorded example of such a triple achievement. Even though Tait recorded the operation some years after the event there is no reason to disbelieve it, for he gave the initials and age of the patient and the doctor's name as identification, and no one ever refuted the report.

This same paper describes a second case operated upon in 1886. This is clearly an example of early and successful removal of an acutely inflamed appendix. It is strange that the third case of appendicitis in this report, operated upon in 1889, was managed by splitting the appendix along its whole length, removing an obstructing calculus and leaving a fine tube as a drain in the opened appendix. In 1889 Tait indicated that he had discarded the idea of removing the appendix, for he published a short report of this third case in that year, remarking that "I have twice in cases similar removed the appendix but am disposed to think that the risk of this operation is somewhat increased by this detail." Although he undoubtedly was far ahead of others in daring to remove the acutely inflamed appendix it cannot be said that he did much to popularise this very sound operation. McKay, perhaps for this reason, does not even mention Tait's work on appendicitis. Had he persisted in his original policy he would have had an even more important "first" to add to his many triumphs. It was left to Fitz and Deaver in the United States to establish the operation from 1890 onwards while British surgeons lagged behind.

The surgery of the kidney was seldom attempted with any frequency before 1870. There were sporadic examples of drainage of abscesses arising from renal disease and occasionally stones were removed fortuitously in the course of such operations. A planned and successful nephrectomy, or removal of the whole kidney, was achieved in 1870 by Gustav Simon (1824-1876) in Germany. Tait stated that he "had seen Simon's case"; it seems likely that on one of his brief visits to Germany he saw the patient after her recovery but that he did not view the operation.

In 1884 Tait reported his first nephrectomy and 11 "nephrotomies"; all the patients recovered. He had been interested in such operations for some time and probably did his first exploration or drainage of a diseased kidney in 1874. The nephrectomy, which he had already reported separately to the annual meeting of the British Medical Association in Worcester in 1882, was an unusual case. In the previous year he had explored an uncertain tumour by the abdominal route, recognised that it was of renal origin but thought it was inoperable. However, a few months later he operated again on this patient—a woman of 24—by a lumbar approach. Unfortunately there is uncertainty about the pathology of the tumour.

By 1889 he had performed 74 operations on the kidney, including 22 nephrectomies with only four deaths. He was well ahead of most of his fellow surgeons in his experience and in his results. His technique varied, for he chose either the lumbar or the anterior abdominal approach according to the circumstances in each case. He usually controlled the large blood vessels of the kidney pedicle with a wire snare, or *serre-noeud*, before removing the organ; the metallic device was extracted a few days later. Tait had, therefore, a part in advancing renal surgery. As early as his student days he had given thought to the possibility of operating on the kidney for different diseases, for in one of his papers he remarks that "it is not twenty years since I was plucked at an examination merely for suggesting that a suppurating kidney, discharging pints of pus into the bladder, should be made to discharge into the loin, or even removed." This was, at the time, a rather daring suggestion for a student to make and it is not surprising that it horrified his examiners!

Tait was also interested in the condition known as "floating kidney" to which many clinicians attributed, usually erroneously, a variety of symptoms and for which (about 1880) a fixation operation or even a nephrectomy was advocated. Tait was vehement in his denunciation of such operations: "I have never yet met with a movable kidney where mobility was the only pathological condition", he wrote. Of the operation for fixation he said in 1893 that he had "narrowly watched the rise and decline of this operation because it is one I distrusted from the first." In fact nephropexy, or fixation of the kidney, continued to be done long after Tait's time, but today it is agreed that it can very seldom be justified; Tait has been proved correct in his evaluation. He was not a urologist, in the modern sense, but inevitably with his gynaecological work he was involved in the diagnosis and management of bladder diseases. Early in his career he advocated a more general use of the direct abdominal approach for operations to remove stones from the bladder.

Tait did not have a very great experience of the management of the common abdominal emergencies arising from acute obstruction of the bowel. In a discussion about 1880 one surgeon complained bitterly that the physicians held these patients and sought the help of the surgeon only as a *"dernier ressort"*. In consequence the results of operation were appalling and a vicious circle developed by which the physician became even more reluctant to hand such cases over to the surgeon.

Tait did encounter examples of intestinal obstruction due to adhesions after procedures such as ovariotomy and he operated on these successfully. He had a little experience of the problems of acute colonic obstruction, usually from malignancy, managed by the formation of a colostomy proximal to the growth. He favoured lumbar colostomy, the technique of which he had learned in Edinburgh from Mackenzie Edwards. He was reluctant to make a colostomy by direct access through the anterior abdominal wall. This was a little surprising in view of his constant preaching on the desirability of direct abdominal section for almost all conditions. If his experience was limited he at least insisted on urgent operation for all obstructions.

Tait was not much involved otherwise in the surgery of gastrointestinal conditions. Gastro-enterostomy (a bypass operation between the stomach and the upper small intestine) was first performed in 1881 and soon became a common procedure. Although Tait recorded no personal experience of this operation he did not hesitate to make rather a foolish criticism for he declaimed that "we know that such operations . . . lead to faecal regurgitation so that the whole scheme of such operations is gradually being dropped." Frederic Treves, who in 1882 was more directly involved in the surgery of the digestive tract, had initially a similar pessimistic view of gastro-enterostomy. It may well be that when the operation was first introduced it was done by some over-enthusiastic and inexperienced surgeons who joined the stomach to the wrong level of the small intestine, with unfortunate effects!

Tait was interested in the surgery of hernia of all kinds. He published quite a large series of successful operations for umbilical hernia in adults. He read a paper, "speaking as a gynaecologist doing incidental herniotomies", at a clinical meeting in 1891 in which he advocated an original mid-line approach to operations for the common types of herniae in the groin. Not surprisingly he was severely criticised by those more experienced in such conditions.

Such were some of his specific contributions in the field of general abdominal surgery. While his work on gallbladder disease was perhaps the most important, it must be emphasised that he exerted his greatest influence by advancing three general ideas. First of all he insisted on early diagnosis and urgent operation for acute abdominal conditions, whether associated with bleeding, obstruction, or infection. Secondly, he overcame the reluctance of his contemporaries to operate in the presence of acute peritonitis. Thirdly, he preached the value of exploratory laparotomy in chronic conditions in which diagnosis was uncertain. Today these ideas are commonplace and accepted without argument; in Tait's time they were revolutionary.

With his experience of ovariotomy it was inevitable that Tait would encounter the relatively frequent acute complication of twisting or torsion of a cyst. It will be recalled that in his Wakefield days he discovered such a condition at an autopsy. He never forgot this case and recalled it in 1879 when he reported his first successful removal of a gangrenous cyst following acute twisting of the pedicle. By 1881 he had had experience of three such cases and in reporting these he discussed the origin of what he now termed "axial rotation". Other surgeons knew of this complication but Tait was one of the first to diagnose it accurately and to appreciate the necessity of urgent intervention. It was this kind of experience which led him on to the success which he achieved in dealing with ruptured ectopic gestation.

It was less easy to find acceptance for urgent operation for acute infective conditions within the abdomen. Tait had for long treated acute pelvic abscess originating from a variety of diseases by urgent drainage through the abdominal approach. Other surgeons tended to withhold surgery for as long as possible, and if they did intervene they preferred to drain the abscess by the vaginal route. In a paper entitled "On the treatment of pelvic suppuration by abdominal section and drainage", read to the Royal Medico-Chirurgical Society in 1880, Tait convinced most of his audience of the merits of his technique by the abdominal approach. In the discussion Erichsen, whose opinion counted greatly, considered that "a new field of surgery had been opened up." Even Spencer Wells supported his rival's views and agreed that now the surgeon had "no dread of peritoneal operations." It was a great advance to overcome the long accepted fear of invading the abdominal cavity in the presence of sepsis.

From his experience of dealing with localised abscesses in the abdominal cavity it was not surprising that Tait soon took the bolder step of operating on patients diagnosed as having general peritonitis. He generously attributed to Alfred Wiltshire (1839-1886) the first deliberate and successful emergency operation for acute peritonitis, in this case due to torsion of an ovarian cyst.[9] Most of Tait's early acute cases of this type, which he first described in 1875, were of peritonitis associated with acute tubal infection. By 1885 he had done 44 such operations with only one death. He attributed his success to early operation and insisted that the septic focus, the inflamed tube or pyosalpinx, should be removed. When Tait claimed some priority in advocating this new principle he came to blows with Frederick Treves who was now becoming prominent as a bold abdominal surgeon. Treves claimed that he had developed this new concept. Once more the matter of priority is unimportant but Tait must be given most of the credit for persuading his contemporaries to discard their cautious approach. It must be conceded that his results were remarkable when it is remembered that he had no antibiotics and none of the refinements of fluid and electrolyte control by intravenous infusion, on which the modern surgeon depends so much.

Tait may not have been the only surgeon to recommend that laparotomy should be a routine diagnostic procedure for chronic abdominal disease of uncertain origin but he was the one who proved that this was a safe and well-justified procedure. He was well aware of the inaccuracy of clinical diagnosis, admitting even his own deficiencies in this respect. His doctrine is summed up in an address he gave in Glasgow in 1891, "On the principle of exploration and confirmatory incisions." He proudly stated that this principle was known as "Tait's law" in America implying, as he frequently did, that a prophet was not honoured in his own country! He had first proposed that there should be a ready use of exploratory laparotomy in 1875. He had to prove that the risks of such operations were acceptable.

It was not surprising that Tait encountered vehement opposition when he first advocated this completely new principle. Most of the opposition came from the London surgeons. In time he convinced them of the relative safety of such procedures, but they feared a "laparotomy epidemic" which might well tempt some to undertake such exploratory operations without real justification. Tait himself saw this danger. His own experience gave ample support to this new conception of abdominal surgery for in 1882, in a series of 208 abdominal sections he did 13 exploratory operations with no deaths. In his survery of his first 1,000 abdominal sections there were 94 such operations with four deaths.

It is relevant to note that modern surgeons are not so ready to apply "Tait's Law" because they have now so many sophisticated diagnostic techniques available to them. However, it is now being realised that there might be some advantage in returning to Tait's conceptions, for there is a tendency to over-investigate patients with abdominal disease, with a consequent delay which may jeopardise the patient's chances of cure and cause needless prolongation of chronic symptoms. In surgery the pendulum swings slowly, and if in some matters Tait has been proved wrong, in others such as this question of diagnosis by early laparotomy, he may well have been right.

His philosophy was expressed very simply in one of his books in 1883 with his supreme and almost arrogant confidence:[10]

> For my own part, so fearless am I now of abdominal surgery, so splendid have been my results in fields of practice, which, until three years ago, seemed hopelessly enclosed that I venture to lay down a surgical law, that in every case of disease in the abdomen or pelvis, in which the health is destroyed or life threatened, and in which the condition is not evidently due to malignant disease, an exploration of the cavity should be made.

He amplified this statement later and clarified a rather pessimistic attitude to malignant disease. "However advanced a case might have been he never refused operation, even when there was a strong reason to suspect malignancy for he made an exploratory incision to remove all doubt."

The details of Tait's operative technique, by which he achieved such outstanding success in gynaecological and general abdominal surgery, are discussed later. His methods were influenced by his attitudes to Lister's introduction of the antiseptic system of surgery, a facet which will be considered in the next chapter (VI). It will be seen that the picture is confused and that there are many contradictions.

CHAPTER VI

Evolution of Antiseptic Surgery and Tait's Opposition to Lister

To assess any surgeon active in the last 30 years of the 19th century his attitudes towards the introduction of the antiseptic system of surgery must be examined. By 1870 very few had accepted Lister's teaching completely; many dabbled in the methods and, without a fair trial, discarded them; some surgeons refused even to give the system any trial. It has been shown that Lawson Tait, while in Wakefield, did employ the antiseptic system but was dissatisfied with his results. He consequently became a most vehement and persistent critic of Lister. To understand Tait's reactions it is relevant to assess further the influence of his teachers in Edinburgh and to look at contemporary controversies, in particular that between those who accepted the germ theory of disease and those who did not.

The decade of the 1860s, which included Tait's student and immediate post-graduate years, was one of extraordinary development both in medicine and general science. Many medical students or young doctors must have encountered teachers who resisted the new ideas. Some confusion may be excused in the minds of most, but the more intelligent would be influenced by the more progressive teachers. Perhaps the average doctor at this time tended to practise what he had been taught at his medical school and was reluctant to alter his ideas or techniques throughout his professional career. There were exceptions, such as Lawson Tait, who retained through their working lives an intense curiosity and an active critical faculty, but even a rebellious individual like Tait remained to some extent under the influence of those teachers who had impressed their views on him in this the most receptive period of his life.

In the general scientific field chemistry had advanced almost explosively. This was reflected in medicine by a rapid increase in the use of qualitative and quantitative tests of the blood or other body fluids or tissues. There was also – as a result of the discoveries of the chemists – the view that even the most basic biological processes could be explained in terms of chemical reactions. Discoveries such as the synthesis of the organic substance urea by Wohler in 1828 supported such ideas. The natural phenomenon of fermentation, which for long had puzzled scientists and philosophers, was considered by the chemists to be explicable on the basis of a chemical process and it is possible that this concept slowed the establishment of a true understanding of biological principles. The cellular theories of life and disease, processes expounded by Virchow, did make a strong impact on pathological teaching and influenced British medicine most markedly in this decade. Despite this influence, aided by the essential if reluctant acceptance of the use of the microscope, improvements in therapeutics were slow to follow. Treatments such as venesection were discarded unwillingly and the traditional use of drugs such as mercury and arsenic, which were highly toxic, was still obstinately practiced. The popularity of homeopathy in Great Britain about this time, however, had a beneficial effect by forcing the orthodox physician to revise his methods.

In the scientific revolution two events of the century cannot be ignored, for their impact on medicine (directly or indirectly) was immense. Firstly, there was the new assessment by the geologists of the age and structure of the earth; secondly, there was the publication in 1859 by Charles Darwin of his work *On the Origin of Species by Means of Natural Selection: or the Preservation of Favoured Races in the Struggle for Life.* Both these new ideas were seen as contrary to the teaching of the Church. It was in the decade from 1860 to 1870 that the argument concerning Darwin's theories were at their height and already the wholesale rejection of the story of the Creation as recounted in Genesis had, from the evidence of the geologists, caused sufficient turmoil.

Before these arguments developed the Established Church had a powerful influence on medicine. In England the Universities of Oxford and Cambridge admitted no non-conformists and the influential College of Physicians was for long ruled by graduates of these two Universities. The hospitals were charitable institutions greatly dominated in their government by the clergy. It has been observed how in Birmingham the early medical school came under excessive influence from the faculty of theology. In London the foundation in 1825 of the "godless" University College and later of its associated teaching hospital was a reaction to such dominance. In Scotland, although there were no sectarian restrictions to the entry of students to the universities, the appointment of professors was biassed in this respect. The vast majority of medical men in the Victorian age were greatly influenced in the conduct of their professional lives by their religious faiths and there was a strong sense of vocation amongst them. While this religious influence can be overstated it cannot be ignored.

For many doctors the mental conflict induced by the new science was extreme and we cannot dismiss the possible influence of this on their philosophies and practice. A few were so convinced of the overthrow of theological dogma that they became avowed agnostics, but many were unable to discard their religious faith. It is difficult to know how often this reluctance stultified the imagination or retarded a career. It is possible that the powerful stream of conservatism, so prominent a feature of 19th century medicine, had its origin in this struggle.[1]

William Lawrence (1763-1857), a rising young surgeon of St. Bartholomew's Hospital, when appointed Professor of Anatomy to the Royal College of Surgeons of England delivered (in 1816) a series of lectures on the "Natural History of Man". In these he showed conclusively that belief in the accuracy of the Biblical account of the Creation was inconsistent with scientific facts. His colleagues were scandalized and John Abernethy, his senior at St. Bartholomew's, accused him of "surrendering the honourable office extended to him by the College of Surgeons to the unworthy desire of propagating opinions detrimental to Society, and of loosening those restraints on which the welfare of mankind depends." Although Lawrence published his lectures he did to some extent recant, only to find himself vilified by free-thinkers as a traitor to the cause of free thought! He was a man of great potential brilliance and rose to considerable eminence. It does appear, however, that his youthful sparks of originality and critical thought were damped by the attacks made upon him, for he contributed little of note to surgery and is remembered mainly as a remarkable orator and a medico-politician.[2]

Dr. Andrew Combe (1797-1847), an Edinburgh physician of some repute, in a letter to a friend concerning the newly published *Vestiges of Creation* by Robert Chambers, wrote these words:[3]

> How creation was effected or according to what laws, is perhaps a question impenetrable by a created being and I feel but little interest in discussing it, because it is at present entirely conjectured. To speculate . . . . on a profound mystery, viz., the beginning of things is an idle employment for beings who have a more practical work placed before them than they can accomplish.

Tait attended a course of lectures in 1862 given by the eminent anatomist, Professor Goodsir. Among other things he heard that:[4]

> . . . . the human body itself is far superior to that of the animal and here I differ from Isadore St. Hilaire and Quatrefois. . . . they both, like Huxley, consider that the body of man is nearer in its structure to the higher ape than the higher ape is to the lower. This I deny, the object of this course is to show the absolute perfection of the human body is a sufficient warrant that man cannot be placed in any zoological series. . . man is a member of the Spiritual Kingdom.
>
> All science properly so called has arisen within the Christian era. One present danger is to elevate science above the other forms of human belief.

It should be noted that Goodsir, in his lectures, made no mention of Darwin and it does seem that for many years Darwinism was unacceptable to most if not all of the Edinburgh professors in the faculties of science and medicine.

There is in the wider field of science a classic account of an individual whose career was very markedly influenced by his reluctance to accept the Darwinian theory. Philip Gosse (1810-1888), a zoologist and marine biologist of distinction, Fellow of the Royal Society in 1856, when faced with the implications of the evolutionary doctrine could not reconcile this with his intense religious beliefs. His son Edmond Gosse writes:[5]

> My father's attitude towards the theory of natural selection was critical in his career . . . . every instinct in his intelligence went out at first to greet the new light. It had hardly done so when a recollection of the opening chapter of Genesis checked it at the outset. He consulted with Carpenter a great investigator but one who was fully as incapable as himself of remodelling his ideas with regard to the old accepted hypothesis. They both determined to have nothing to do with the terrible theory, but to hold steadily to the law of the fixity of species.

Philip Gosse published a book in which he defended his attitude, suggesting that the Creator had planted prefabricated fossils in the rocks to test the faith of man! Thereafter he made few significant contributions to science and his promising career was cut short.

The doctors were not in the vanguard of those who participated in the arguments over Darwinism. This may be explained in light of the fact that relatively few were involved in pure research or scientific studies. The epidemologist Benjamin Babington remarked that "The great majority of medical practitioners are so fully engaged in practical medicine that they have little time left for the more searching and scientific enquiries which we profess to undertake." Thomas Huxley was more explicit when he expressed a very low opinion of the scientific basis of contemporary medicine.

It is now pertinent to review the development of understanding of the germ theory of disease, for clearly much of the antagonism to Lister's ideas arose from the failure of so many surgeons to understand or accept this concept. This cannot be discussed without allusion to the theory of spontaneous generation.

While in Biblical and other early writings the idea of the spread of disease by contagion or contact is remarkably clearly expressed, it is to Girolamo Frascatorius (1478-1553) that we owe an account of the transmission of infective diseases which, for the time, was remarkably practical.[6] Frascatorius differentiated three possible modes of infection: contagion by direct personal contact, contagion by contact with fomites (clothes or other articles touched by diseased persons), and contagion at a distance. He wrote of the "seminaria" of disease, but to translate this as "germs" is incorrect, for he may have implied anything from a smell or "exhalation" to the transmission of particles of indeterminate matter. He recognised the possibility of airborne infection, the environmental risks in consumption, the direct inoculation of hydrophobia by the bite of a rabid dog, the mode of transmission of syphilis, and he knew much about the natural history of epidemics of plague and typhus. Much of what Frascatorius taught was soon forgotten and had to be rediscovered. His possible conception of "seminaria" as the germs of disease was revived with the development of the microscope in the seventeenth century. Anton van Leeuwenhoek (1632-1723) was amongst the first to demonstrate with a crude microscope a world of micro-organisms or living animalcula. That these could be associated with disease processes soon became the subject of much philosophical argument but it was from indirect studies that a fully substantiated germ theory of disease was developed.

For long the natural phenomenon of fermentation, as seen in the making of bread, wine, or beer, had mystified men. It was not until the 19th century that the elucidation of such processes laid the foundation of the science of bacteriology. This, unlike most other sciences, started as an applied science without a basic scientific discipline. Early bacteriologists were more interested in the effects of micro-organisms, whether in relation to industrial techniques or to disease processes, than in the precise way they functioned as living creatures.

In 1836 Cagniard-Latour described clearly how yeast consisted of living cells reproducing by budding and causing the breakdown of sugars into carbonic acid and alcohol. This new biological theory of fermentation, developed further by Schwann and Kützing, was not accepted by most contemporary scientists, who believed that this process as well as the basic phenomena of life could be explained on the basis of the interaction of chemical processes. Chemists such as Berzelius, Liebig and Wöhler strongly opposed Cagniard-Latour's conception of the action of yeast. It remained for Louis Pasteur (1822-1895), by his meticulous experimental work and his "fanatic's zeal to force his conviction on the world", to establish beyond question the validity of the biological process involved in fermentation. He identified the micro-organisms which caused the "diseases" [*i.e.*, changes] in wines. It is noteworthy that he used the term "diseases", which reflected his early belief that studies in this specialized field of bacteriology could in time be applied to the elucidation and control of human ailments.

Pasteur showed from his experiments that fermentation in wine or milk was caused by micro-organisms and was not a chemical process. In countless experiments he proved that a sterilised broth would not undergo fermentation or putrefaction if entry of air was prevented. He showed that the air of crowded cities was laden with dust particles on which micro-organisms were carried, while pure air at high altitudes was relatively germ-free. He also proved that the processes of fermentation were actuated by organisms found in the atmosphere. To extend the germ theory of fermentation to a germ theory of disease was the next step.

It was inevitable that there should soon have been attempts to apply Pasteur's discoveries and techniques to the elucidation and management of infected wounds. There had long been an association in the minds of many doctors between the phenomena of fermentation and the process of wound infection (or putrefaction). Joseph Lister (1827-1912) had for some years thought deeply about the origin of infection of wounds. He had moved from Edinburgh when appointed to the Chair of Surgery in Glasgow in 1860. The incidence of hospital infection was higher in the Glasgow Infirmary than in the Edinburgh Infirmary. The wards in which he worked in Glasgow were built over a cemetery in which thousands of victims of a cholera epidemic had been buried in shallow graves. In this somewhat unfavourable environment Lister was to achieve his remarkable success in the management of compound fractures by a new technique.

From his earlier days with Syme in Edinburgh Lister had studied the healing of wounds and the reaction of tissues to injury. He had concluded that "suppuration in wounds is decomposition, brought about by the influence of the atmosphere upon blood or serum retained within them. . . ." Like others he had pondered deeply over the question as to why a simple fracture without an external wound did not become septic, while a compound fracture almost invariably did so. He had experimented with many dressing techniques and with numerous antiseptic substances. The term "antiseptic" had long been used: as early as 1751 John Pringle, an Army surgeon, had described substances which resisted or promoted putrefaction in wounds as either "antiseptic" or "septic". Amongst the antiseptics already in common use was carbolic acid, applied to wounds or ulcers empirically and without understanding of its mode of action.

It is curious that Lister did not know of Pasteur's discoveries until early in 1865 when Thomas Anderson, Professor of Chemistry in Glasgow, drew his attention to the French chemist's work in a chance conversation. Pasteur's original papers were, of course, in French scientific periodicals to which Lister may not have had ready access, but there *were* comments in British medical periodicals long before 1865. The *British Medical Journal* in 1861 had a brief annotation on "The Cause of fermentation", referring to Pasteur's discovery that this process was caused by "infusoria" or "vibrios".[7] In 1862 a brief report was made on Pasteur's description of the destructive action of micro-organisms in wounds.[8] More significant were two prominent leaders in the *Journal* in 1862 entitled "The Fermentative Theory of disease".[9] The anonymous author of these leaders deserves some credit for drawing attention to Pasteur's work in detail and for having the perspicacity to state that "the discoveries made by this savant concerning the organic corpuscles contained in the air furnish us with certain theoretical and practical facts worthy of consideration in relation to the etiology of purulent infection." The writer referred to the eminent French doctor Anton Trousseau (1801-1867 who in his lectures had discussed the parallel of fermentation and wound putrefaction. Trousseau believed that micro-organisms might be deposited in the body, in an open wound for example, to act locally or to cause general effects and that the diseases of "hospital gangrene, malignant pustules and contagious erysipelas" could be caused in this way. He also suggested that the infectious material might be conveyed "by the air or by the dressings." A final paragraph from Trousseau's teaching deserves quotation, for it embodies ideas which in time were to be substantiated:

> These germs will not be developed as readily in all patients. Some patients, like certain earths will not receive the same seeds . . . . the soil may be too wet, there too dry, here other germs have grown up and stifled the new seed. Just so is it not with morbid germs and ferments? They individually require conditions favourable to their development.

Trousseau had developed his argument to ascribe wound infection to airborne organisms, the same argument which Lister was to evolve from Pasteur's work. For treatment Trousseau advocated cauterisation of wounds to kill the organisms and to seal off the raw tissue. He suggested also that ligatures carried infection into wounds. The annotator ended by emphasising that these ideas were merely speculative "but we recommend them to the consideration of the profession." There was no comment on these articles in the correspondence columns; however, at least one surgeon—Spencer Wells—seems to have taken note of them. In August 1864, at the annual meeting of the British Medical Association held in Cambridge, Spencer Wells contributed a paper entitled "Some causes of excessive mortality after surgical operations."[10] He showed that he was completely familiar with Pasteur's work. He recounted each relevant experiment, explained how Pasteur had proved that airborne micro-organisms initiated fermentation processes and described these micro-organisms in detail. He accepted the germ theory of disease and was satisfied that Pasteur had demolished the theory of spontaneous generation. He affirmed that Pasteur's work offered an understanding of the "influence of atmospheric germs upon our bodies in health and disease." Wells knew also of Calvert (whose work had been noted in the *British Medical Journal* of 1862). This Frenchman had shown that micro-organisms could be found in septic dressings and in the grime and dust on hospital walls. Wells was also aware of the suggestion of Davaine in 1850 that there was a specific bacterial infection in animals affected with the "carbuncular disease" of "splenic apoplexy", namely anthrax.

Wells had grasped the explanation of wound infection but did not conceive, as Lister was soon to do, a technique which could be applied practically to surgery. Instead he diverted in his paper to the work of Polli of Italy, who accepted the notion that the general effects of pyaemia were caused by micro-organisms in the blood and treated such conditions by chemotherapy in the form of various sulphites. Wells had tried hyposulphite of soda given orally and he believed it had some value. He dismissed the more pressing problem of prevention against wound infection by insisting merely on his own "scrupulous purity and cleanliness" in surgical technique.

There was a discussion about this paper, but no one commented directly on Pasteur's discoveries. Routh knew about the "spores" which might cause infection, but he was rather ignorant about their size, for he thought he could keep them out of the wards by having perforated zinc screens on the windows! Thudichum made the sensible suggestion that dirty dressings should be burned. Camps thought that a lavish dose of opium was the answer to all the problems of infection! Radclyffe Hall believed that if ward ventilation was improved by open fireplaces the dreaded germs would be sucked away. No one seems to have grasped the whole picture which Spencer Wells presented so clearly.

Although he was a member of the Association, Lister was not at the Cambridge meeting. It is a little surprising that he did not read Wells' paper when it was published in both the *British Medical Journal* and the *Lancet* in September 1864, for it was on a subject in which he was already intensely interested. There is evidence however that he was not an avid reader of the writings of others, preferring to work out his own ideas and submit them to his own painstaking experimental research.

Besides Trousseau and Wells there were others before 1865 who looked critically at Pasteur's discoveries. John Hughes Bennet (1812-1879), Professor of the Institutes of Medicine in Edinburgh, delivered a lecture on "Atmospheric germ theory" to the Royal College of Surgeons of Edinburgh early in 1868, in which he revealed that since 1863 he had begun a series of observations after reading Pasteur's papers.[11] He repeated many of Pasteur's experiments, with different results. He studied with great care the micro-organisms which developed in his cultures. From his own observations he supported the view of Pouchet that the "infusoria" or organisms which appeared to grow in a sealed vessel developed in a "finely molecular pellicle on the surface of decomposing fluids without pre-existing cells or germs and independently of parents." Bennet drew a series of diagrams of a variety of organisms developing from indeterminate "molecules" which had coalesced to form chained structures (rather like the streptococci which we recognise today) or "vibrios" (rod-like organisms) with motility and with the power of reproduction by division. As far as we can ascertain he had no technique of staining these organisms to show them clearly, but instead depended on the interpretation of the rather ghostly shadows of untreated material. Meticulous though Bennet's drawings are we are forced to the conclusion that this sequence of illustrations was made to some extent to fit a theory in which he had implicit belief. Although his experiments involved a careful technique to prevent the entry of the outside air to his flasks, it seems probable that there were errors similar to those which Pouchet had made and to which Pasteur eventually drew attention. Nevertheless it is of some interest that while Tait was a student in Edinburgh there was at least one worker in this new field. Perhaps Tait heard Bennet lecture on the subject; certainly he recorded later how greatly he had been influenced by the molecular theory. It is a little surprising that in the relatively close medical community of Edinburgh Lister apparently did not know of Bennet's interest in the work of Pasteur.

However belatedly and fortuitously he heard of Pasteur's discoveries Lister seized upon them brilliantly. Thanks to his father's instruction (Joseph Jackson Lister was a skilled microscopist who had developed the achromatic lens) he could appreciate the techniques which Pasteur had employed. Lister also knew something (his father was a wine merchant) of the phenomenon of fermentation. More significantly, Lister had done experimental work in his early years on the pathology of inflammation. Thus he had what Pasteur referred to as the "prepared mind", by which a scientist could grasp the significance of some simple and apparently unrelated clue or idea with reference to a major problem.

Before he read Pasteur's description of airborne micro-organisms, Lister had already suspected that if in some way he could protect a wound from contact with the air he could do much to prevent infection or putrefaction in wounds. Many before him had entertained similar ideas. When Lister became aware of the true nature of the infecting agent in the air, the method became logical and its application practical. It was this immediate awareness of the significance of micro-organisms in wound infection that revealed Lister's genius. Initially he concentrated on Pasteur's teaching that "every speck of dust carries at least one germ." Soon he realised that the contamination of wounds by soil or road dust, by dirty instruments, by dirty ligatures and by the unwashed hands of the surgeon were other potent sources of infection. Many others – Syme, Simpson and Semmelweiss for example – had already grasped individual points, but it was Lister who was the first to see the whole picture clearly and to relate it to Pasteur's theories. He knew that Syme had achieved good results in his surgical practice by insisting on scrupulous cleanliness of hands and instruments, a most unusual precaution amongst his contemporaries. If Lister had read Simpson's book on acupressure he would have appreciated the fact that unclean ligatures were a likely source of trouble and that to leave dead tissue in the depths of a wound was often calamitous. Simpson had sent Lister a copy of his book in 1865 with a letter expressing the hope that Lister would accept it:[12]

> To my "medical mind" it appears most strange and inexplicable that surgeons do go on sedulously and systematically implanting by the ligature two, four, six or more fragments of dead and decomposing arterial tissue in every large wound and yet say they wish these wounds to heal by first intention. . . . It is the stranger when all late experience has proved that the needle is at least as effectual a haemostatic as the ligature.

Simpson's book on acupressure was much more than the exposition of his special technique, for it embodied a study of wound healing in which he established many principles which are accepted today.

Like most surgeons, Lister does not appear to have known initially of the work of Semmelweiss who (as early as 1846) had cut down the incidence of fatal puerperal sepsis in his wards by the simple expedient of insisting that all attendants on patients should wash their hands in an antiseptic solution.[13] It was one great jigsaw puzzle and in Pasteur's work Lister recognised the last piece and put it in place.

Lister had to choose a substance which would destroy micro-organisms but which could be applied safely and conveniently in his operating and dressing techniques. Pasteur had used heat as a sterilising agent in his experiments, boiling his solutions and flaming his instruments. In fact, he flamed his hands prior to some of his manipulations! Excessive heat could not, of course, be applied to living tissues. Lister wanted to achieve two things. Firstly, germs must be prevented from getting into wounds during and after planned operations and, if possible, they must be killed outside the wound also. Secondly, if germs had already entered an accidental wound—as in a compound fracture before the case was seen by him—these germs must be washed out of the wound or killed before they had time to spread. He had already tried many of the known antiseptic substances. Before he appreciated the germ theory of disease he had used carbolic acid in his dressing techniques. This he continued to use, for when he became aware of Pasteur's work he heard of the successful employment of the crude oil as a "disinfectant" to kill certain parasites which infected cattle grazing on pasture contaminated by sewage. He was often to make the point that he might well have chosen another antiseptic and found it equally effective. Many problems arose from his choice of carbolic acid, not least of which was that of calculation of the strength and purity of his solutions so that the maximum bactericidal effect might be achieved with minimum danger to live tissues. Despite all problems, between 1865 and 1867 he evolved a technique that produced the dramatic results which he published in the *Lancet.*[14]

When Lister introduced his antiseptic technique using carbolic acid he was immediately accused of plagiarism, and indeed this accusation has never completely died down. The only plagiarism suggested was in his use of carbolic acid as an antiseptic substance. In 1863 Jules Lemaire (1814- ?) had published *De l'Acide Phénique,* followed by a second edition in 1865. It was well before 1860 that it was known that coal tar derivatives, including carbolic acid, had a powerful "disinfectant" action on chronic ulcers and septic wounds. Following the discovery of means of purifying preparations of carbolic acid, Lemaire – a skilled pharmacist as well as a physician – undertook clinical studies involving the use of carbolic acid dressings. Despite a flat denial of the efficacy of such treatment by the influential surgeon Velpeau, Lemaire continued his research and, more importantly, was convinced by 1862 that Pasteur's discoveries could be applied to surgery. As early as 1860 he had proved to his satisfaction that carbolic acid acted by destroying micro-organisms of various types. By 1865, in the second edition of his book, he expressed the view that micro-organisms in the pus of infected wounds were killed off by carbolic acid. Lemaire's discovery was strangled at its birth, largely by the conservative surgeons who dominated Paris at the time. Lemaire gave up his studies and so "faded from the pages of medical history." He wrote with resignation, "Happy am I if I have been able to attain the goal which is my sole ambition – to be useful . . . . I am but a simple artisan who buys material to construct an edifice that architects more skilful than I shall complete."[15] Lister was to be the architect.

It was Simpson who first drew Lister's attention to Lemaire's work. A few weeks after the Dublin meeting at which Lister elaborated on the technique he had already published in the *Lancet*, Simpson wrote to the *Edinburgh Daily Review* under the pseudonym of "Chirurgicus", stating that Lister's writings were "calculated to bring down upon us discredit—particularly among our French and German neighbours—insofar as it attributes the first surgical employment of carbolic acid to Professor Lister of Glasgow. . . ." Simpson had read Lemaire's book, for there was a copy in the Edinburgh University Library, and he knew that Lemaire had demonstrated the power of carbolic acid to destroy micro-organisms. Shortly afterwards Simpson published a long article in the *Lancet* accusing Lister of claiming an undeserved priority.[16] There was some justification for Simpson's article, but it was unfortunately a somewhat bigoted personal attack couched in terms which revealed his disappointment that his ideas about acupressure and hospitalism had been rejected and that Lister had stolen his thunder. Lister resented these attacks, particularly the anonymous letter. He replied almost contemptuously:[17]

> The elaborate communication of Sir James Young Simpson in today's Lancet may seem to require some reply. But as I have already endeavoured to place the matter in its true light without doing injustice to anyone, I must forbear from any comment on his allegations.

Lister, who was always fair about matters of priority, went at once to Edinburgh to take out Lemaire's book from the Library. He read it but did not think that Lemaire had evolved a surgical technique which in any way approached his own application of the germ theory of disease. He wrote to the *Lancet:*[18]

> I have seen Dr. Lemaire's work on carbolic acid and find that, where he speaks of the application of that substance, the principles and practice which he mentions are such as sufficiently to explain the results.
>
> I may repeat that I have never claimed to have been the first to use carbolic acid. . . . And I may take the opportunity of warning your readers that they must not expect carbolic acid to work like a charm. . . .

Simpson's attack was unfortunate, for it had the effect of concentrating too much attention on the use of carbolic acid in the antiseptic system of treatment at the expense of an appreciation of the whole theory behind its application. It is interesting to note that James Syme saw the danger of such a misunderstanding, for he wrote to Lister early in 1869: "Instead of 'antiseptic' I think you should call the system of treatment 'protective' to avoid confusion. . . ."[19]

Lemaire should not be forgotten; prior to Lister he had come nearer to the truth than had anyone else. One of Tait's favourite quotations was from Sydney Smith: "It is not the man who first says a thing who deserves the credit, but he who says it so long and so loud that at last he persuades the world it is true." On the same theme the medical historian Charles Singer comments:[20]

> There is, in truth, no such thing as a method of discovery. It may come to one man after immense systematic analysis, to another by analogy, to a third as a sudden thought or vision, to yet another as a dream, and in a hundred other ways. It is demonstration that is the basis of science.

In retrospect it is at first astonishing that Lister's demonstrations were not immediately accepted by all surgeons. He encountered great opposition for many years and some contemporaries never accepted his views. To understand Lawson Tait's battle with Lister it is necessary to appreciate the fact that Tait was not alone in his rejection of this momentous discovery. We may dismiss those critics who acted from an antipathy towards anything new, and Tait can hardly be included in this category! We may forget the critics actuated in part by personal feelings or jealousy. In this category we must regrettably include Sir James Simpson and we could be tempted to place Tait in this group also, but this would be to reject his undoubted ability and his intensive study of the problem. The reactions of the majority can be traced in the medical periodicals of the decade after 1867. The evidence to be found in the *British Medical Journal* is as relevant as any insofar as British surgeons are concerned.

Lister was persuaded to give a paper at the annual meeting of the Association in Dublin in August 1867. The paper was published in the *Journal*, but the editor did not think it worth-while to record the discussion which followed.[21] Yet the annual meeting had become a forum for the expression of new ideas and afforded much publicity to audiences which included the influential leaders of the profession. At each annual meeting there were retrospective and prospective surveys of the state of Medicine in the President's Oration and in the addresses to the different sections of the meeting. At Dublin none of the leading speakers commented on Lister's work, despite the fact that it had been published earlier that year. Next year in Oxford the President, Henry Acland, dismissed the topic in one sentence- "The observations of Pasteur are connected with questions of infection, nay more of suppuration and (as shown probable by Professor Lister) of surgical treatment." This short statement was not perhaps too surprising, for Acland was a physician and still believed firmly in the theory of spontaneous generation. At the same meeting Sir James Paget in the address to the Section of Surgery did not even mention Lister and no papers were offered on any experience of the antiseptic method.

In 1869 the Association came to Leeds for what was to prove to be an important meeting. A symposium on hospital planning, to which Sir James Simpson was to contribute, was arranged and it was inevitable that reference would be made in discussion to the influence of Listerism on the control of hospital infection. It was known in advance that Thomas Nunneley (1809-1870), a well-known Leeds surgeon, would deliver a major attack on Lister in his address to the surgical section. Simpson wrote to Nunneley a month before the meeting.[22]

> How is your address developing itself? I wish anxiously to get up to Leeds to hear it and three papers on the list about Construction of Hospitals and Hospitalism. But I fear that I shall not be able to escape. The Countess of Kintore has come here to have a child . . . . and to have chloroform which her London doctors some years ago refused to give. If she is better in time I will run off; if not I am fixed here.

Simpson went on to summarise the statistics he was going to produce to prove his own theories about the dangers of doing major surgery in large hospitals and gave some illustrations of his success with acupressure and "*no* carbolic acid." The titled patient did well and Simpson was able to come to Leeds. He joined in the discussion on hospital design, the last major occasion on which he expressed his view on hospitalism and his firm belief that the technique of acupressure was much more important than Lister's antisepsis. He was probably delighted with Nunneley's paper.

This time Lister was not ignored. He became, indeed, the target of a lengthy condemnation of his antiseptic system:[23]

> I refer to the recent – shall I venture to say fashionable? – method of treating wounds by what has been called the "antiseptic treatment" by the advocates of which, it is to be feared, the sound physiological and pathological doctrines and practice or the last generation of British surgeons are unheeded. . . . Had the works of John Hunter

been now so generally studied as they once were and the doctrines which he enunciated been carefully kept in mind this fallacy could hardly have obtained the temporary currency it had done.

Such was the tone of Nunneley's speech, which establishes him in the categories of the obstinate and the ultra-conservative. He had failed to understand the germ theory of disease and still supported the idea of spontaneous generation. He admitted that he had never tried Lister's methods, and he misquoted the experience of some of his colleagues in Leeds who had achieved some success with the new technique. But his remarks, however vague, were influential.

Lister did not attend the Leeds meeting; he did, however, reply to Nunneley's accusations with patience and dignity. In a letter to the *Journal* shortly after the meeting he appended a report from Teale, a colleague of Nunneley, who had achieved excellent results with Lister's methods. Lister deplored the fact that Nunneley "should dogmatically oppose a treatment which he so little understands and which by his own admission he has not tried. . . ."[24] There were letters from other surgeons about the address, which expressed more support than criticism of what Nunneley had said. In general the picture in 1869 was one of antagonism to Lister; if here and there some support was given it was only by approval of carbolic acid as a dressing material, but almost completely without acceptance or understanding of the ideas behind the method – and, in particular, of the germ theory of disease. Only one truly relevant paper was given: "On the anti-septic cere-cloth for dressings", delivered by Edward Lund (1823-1898), a Manchester surgeon who at this time was one of Lister's few ardent disciples.

At Newcastle in 1870 a local surgeon by the name of George Heath (1820-1892) addressed the Section in Surgery; he referred briefly but at least a little more favourably to the antiseptic system, and pleaded for less ill-informed prejudice against it. That year there was only one rather insignificant paper relating to Listerism – "Ligature of the femoral: using Lister's plan".

At Plymouth in 1871 Lister himself was invited to address the Section of Surgery. Now it appeared he had the opportunity to convince his critics. He was not entirely successful, although he went through all the details of the method and expounded on the theory from his more recent experimental work. Perhaps many in his audience were still ill-equipped to follow his reasoning. He had doubts himself about his success in convincing them, for he ended his very lengthy and detailed paper rather wearily:[25]

> After statements of this conclusive character have been published regarding what is generally admitted as the most urgent medical question of the day, when I consider the apathy with which they have been received in many quarters, I cannot avoid being reminded of the language of Macbeth –
>
> "Can such things be,
> And overcome us like a summer cloud,
> Without a special wonder?"

If further proof of such apathy were needed it was supplied by Sir William Fergusson, the doyen of London surgeons, who ignored completely the antiseptic system in his Surgical Address at Birmingham the following year (1872). Another year later, when Fergusson was serving as President of the Section of Surgery, he again ignored Lister and his work in his opening speech. However, John Wood of Kings College did give a paper on the antiseptic treatment which was favourable, though hedged about with caution: he did not feel justified "to attempt to discuss atmospheric germs." Among other papers on the subject, Lund of Manchester, under the title of "Fallacies and Failures in Antiseptic Surgery", made a strong plea to surgeons to follow Lister's instructions more meticulously if they hoped to achieve success. Lund's remarks were followed by a lively discussion from which it was all too clear that the London surgeons in particular were still against Lister. One attributed Lister's undoubted success to "general medical and hygienic treatment, rather than the niceties and complexities of his Special System."

In 1874 at Norwich William Cadge affirmed that there was "one great subject waiting for solution, the germ theory of disease", but to his mind any further discussion was useless. In Edinburgh in 1875 Professor James Spence (1812-1882) gave the Address in Surgery and was lukewarm in his support of Lister, preferring the simple methods he had learnt from Syme. But Spence was rather backward in his ideas; he was still a strong advocate of bloodletting. Lister's contribution to this meeting was a paper entitled "The effect of the antiseptic treatment upon the general salubrity of Surgical Hospitals." He listed the acceptance of his principles by surgeons abroad – Saxtorph in Denmark, Nussbaum, Volkmann and Von Langenbeck in Germany, and many others. It was a pointed rebuke to British surgeons.

So it went at these annual conventions. As late as 1879 William Savory (1826-1895) of St. Bartholomew's Hospital made a massive attack on Lister in his address "On the prevention of Blood-poisoning in the practice of surgery."[26] He not only rejected the germ theory but also accused Lister of never having produced comparative statistics to prove that his methods were superior to others.

If such annual appraisals do not reveal adequately the general reluctance to accept Lister's work and the complete failure of so many to understand what it was all about, the evidence can be augmented by a perusal of the ordinary papers appearing in the medical journals during these years. Few writers supported Lister, and even those who did so expressed reservations.

In 1876 Hector Cameron (1843-1928), assistant to Lister in Glasgow, reported success in the management of compound injuries of the knee joint by the antiseptic method but made no mention of bacterial infection. Sir Thomas Smith (1833-1909) of St. Bartholomew's Hospital found the method "sound in the chemical sense but pathologically it may be unsound." A contemporary leader in the *British Medical Journal* on the antiseptic system "equals it with Paget's treatment of pyaemia by keeping the patient in a current of air." This was simply to blow away the dreaded germs; it was hardly a fair comparison! An almost complete lack of understanding is shown by the titles of most of the early papers: instead of the "antiseptic system of surgery", discussion centered on the "carbolic acid treatment of wounds." As late as 1875 the *Lancet* carried leaders which confused the general situation:[27]

> Mr. Lister and his disciples are themselves to blame for much of the obscurity that overshadows this question inasmuch as they have not yet openly and fairly met the challenges . . . . to produce statistical results of their practice . . . . at present less antiseptic surgery is practised in metropolitan hospitals than ever there was.

Lister's move to London in 1877 was in the nature of a crusade, and not without results. About 1880 he had begun to convert the London surgeons to his ideas, at least to some degree. By this time, however, with the general improvement in hospital hygiene and a more ready acceptance of strict cleanliness in technique by most surgeons, the more complicated details of the original antiseptic methods were becoming modified and there was a movement in all countries towards the aseptic technique of surgery.

We may wonder why Lister had so much difficulty getting his ideas accepted. It is clear that there were many reasons. We have commented on the general attitude of conservatism amongst surgeons. Few had the scientific background of Lister, the facility to examine a problem in depth, or minds equipped to progress from a hypothesis through experimental observations to an exact conclusion. Two other aspects require examination. Firstly, granting that Lister's audience was perhaps poorly equipped to grasp the revolutionary conception which he offered, were there in fact deficiencies in his evidence and reasoning which made the acceptance of his case less likely? Secondly, were Lister's colleagues bewildered by the argument which raged concerning the theory of spontaneous generation? This latter controversy had much relevance to the acceptance or rejection of the germ theory of disease.

It is customary to suggest that Lister offered clear-cut evidence to support his case. If we study his original papers today it may seem that this is so; however, *we* read his writings with the advantage of hindsight. If there are gaps in the evidence we too readily fill these in from present knowledge. There are some curious features about Lister's early papers which are surprising in view of his critical approach and his meticulous methods. When Lister read his paper at Dublin in 1867 Sir James Simpson said in a discussion:[28]

> One of the chief reasons for recommending carbolic acid . . . has been that there may be sporules, germs, or fungi floating in the atmosphere, which, if allowed access to the wound would cause irritation and suppuration. No one has yet seen these mystical fungi with the eye or the microscope. . . .

Simpson was incorrect in suggesting that micro-organisms in the atmosphere had not been seen but the implication that Lister himself had not seen such organisms in infected wounds was perhaps justified. It would have been much more convincing had Lister been able to complete his argument by proving that the airborne micro-organisms were in fact to be found in septic wounds. It is true that staining methods to demonstrate the presence of bacteria were crude in the extreme in 1867 but there were already some ideas about culturing infected matter and transmitting organisms from one animal to another. It is surprising that Lister did not even suggest in his early papers that he would like to prove that the presence of specific micro-organisms could be demonstrated in infected wounds. Instead, he merely accepted a current and rather vague theory of pan-spermism by which it was assumed that micro-organisms of various shapes and sizes were merely varieties of one species that took up different forms in response to their environment. Furthermore, Lister made the categorical statement in 1867 that the inflammation associated with an acute abscess was caused by tension and that only when the pus was released did organisms enter the cavity. He did say that "in rare and exceptional cases" organisms were present, and he did record (rather vaguely) that he *had* seen one abscess with pus containing "vibrios". However, he insisted for some years that acute abscesses were sterile until they were opened and made no real attempt to prove this statement, which was erroneous and somewhat misleading.[29] Even in 1880 Lister was reluctant to discard the theory of John Hunter that nervous irritation or "sympathy" was the cause of the signs and symptoms of inflammation, for Lister believed in counter-irritation as an effective treatment. He had remained convinced of the efficacy of Syme's treatment of acutely inflamed joints by the red-hot cautery. It was not that he lacked expertise in bacteriological methods, for he later completed a study of the lactic acid bacillus, an investigation still regarded today as one of the most elaborate and able of any such research in the early history of the science of bacteriology. It is certainly surprising that he did not concentrate his attention on the bacteriology of infected wounds and acute abscesses at the start of his research. Watson Cheyne, one of Lister's London assistants, records that up to the middle of the seventies little work was done on the bacteriology of infected wounds. In the first Lister Memorial Lecture Cheyne recalled that in later years Lister "did occasionally look at the discharges from wounds microscopically", but that initially "the results of his treatment were his test and the success of it seemed to confirm his theories."

At heart Lister was a scientist. Many, such as Sir Charles Sherrington (1857-1952), have commented on Lister's love of research for its own sake and on his achievements in physiology and pathology rather than in the clinical sphere.[30] This was at least one of the reasons why his inaugural address in London in 1877 did not greatly further his cause, for he talked at length about his original and ingenious work by which he had proved that the lactic acid bacillus was the cause of fermentation in milk. This did not impress the London surgeons who still did not see the relevance of such work to their practice.

All through this preliminary period it was clearly the failure of surgeons to appreciate or accept the germ theory of disease, which did much to delay the full acceptance of Lister's teaching. Joseph Bell in Edinburgh accepted the antiseptic technique and practised it with a strict adherence to details; nevertheless he wrote in 1869 that "the existence of germs has at times been affirmed and at times denied. I have no intention to discuss the contention at all nor do I really care whether their existence be granted me or not."[31] Bell was voicing a negative attitude which persisted for long in the minds of most surgeons. Again in 1875 the author of a leader in the *Lancet* suggested that any reduction in the incidence of wound infection thought to be due to the "carbolic acid treatment" was really the result of improvement in the hygiene of hospitals and that "the germ theory may be perfectly well-founded but nine surgeons out ot ten do not care whether it is or not."[32]

To an appreciable extent the reluctance of so many surgeons to accept the germ theory of disease was due to the persistent belief in the theory of spontaneous generation. When Pasteur came on the scene he had to combat this belief that life could be generated *de novo.* Admittedly extravagant propositions, such as that of Von Helmont in the 16th century that mice could be created from a bundle of dirty rags, had been discarded. Redi had shown in the late 17th century that a form of worm, hitherto believed to be hatched spontaneously from decomposing meat, was in fact the larva from an egg laid by a fly alighting on the meat. Spallanzini about 1770 did experiments by which he showed that if he subjected putrescible fluids to prolonged heat he could prevent the growth of "living germs". This weakened support for the theory of spontaneous generation. Pasteur scrutinised all the experiments of those who supported the concept of spontaneous generation of micro-organisms. By perfecting his techniques of filtering the air and sterilising his equipment he demolished his opponents' ideas. Between 1860 and 1864 a controversy between Pasteur and Pouchet, the most vociferous believer in spontaneous generation, reached a peak and was the subject of a public debate in the French Academy. It had to be admitted that Pasteur carried the day. In Great Britain meanwhile Hughes Bennet, as we have noted, was a firm supporter of the theory of spontaneous generation of micro-organisms.

The argument between Pouchet and Pasteur deserves rather closer attention. It is almost invariably stated that Pasteur's case was foolproof and that his concise methodology and meticulous experiments enabled him to crush the more metaphysical approach of Pouchet. In 1859 the latter published his *Hétérogenie, ou traité de la génération spontanie.* In the preface he wrote, "when by meditation it was evident to me that spontaneous generation was one of the means employed by nature for the reproduction of living things, I applied myself to discover the methods by which this takes place." This statement was always to be taken against him as implying that his theories were largely coloured by religious and philosophic views. Pouchet, in fact, was a meticulous experimentalist. He believed that spontaneous generation was by heterogenesis or the development of new life from biological debris or organic matter. He did not accept the idea that spontaneous generation could arise from inorganic matter—the abiogenesis of other theorists. The idea of spontaneous generation had initially been supported by the theologians, but was denounced by the 19th century as heretical and equated with materialism. When Clemence Royer translated Darwin's *Origin of Species* into French in 1861 she attacked the Roman Catholic Church in her introduction to the book. It was the era of the Third Empire, a government reactionary to revolutionary thought and linked closely with the Catholic hierarchy. Pouchet entered the lists with inevitable opposition from the Académie des Sciences, a body which largely supported current political and theological ideas.[33]

In 1862 the Academy appointed a commission to award a prize of 2,500 francs "to him who, by well conducted experiments throws new light on the question of so-called spontaneous generation." The commission was heavily biassed against Pouchet who, realising this, withdrew from the competition. The prize was awarded to Pasteur. Two years later a new commission was appointed to re-examine the question; again there was support for Pasteur, without fair consideration of Pouchet's arguments.

When he was involved in these arguments Pasteur, in fact, was engaged in a series of experiments aimed at establishing the possibility of spontaneous generation of life. He was conducting elaborate chemical experiments based on his theory of "asymetric forces", which he had developed from his brilliant work on the optical activity of crystalline substances. But he kept remarkably quiet about this aspect of his work and it has been suggested that in his attack on Pouchet he was greatly influenced by political and theological considerations. It was written of Pasteur that "he did not permit his religious convictions to influence his scientific conclusions" and that "his canon, as a scientist . . . was to stand aloof from religion, philosophy, materialism and spiritualism." There are grounds for applying such statements more justifiably to Pouchet. In later life Pasteur, an intensely patriotic Frenchman, denounced certain German discoveries in bacteriology not from an unbiassed scientific scrutiny but because the Germans had inflicted such damage on his beloved France in the Franco-Prussian War. In 1872, when the theory of spontaneous generation still persisted in some quarters, he described it as German in origin and said that no patriotic Frenchman would support it.

We have digressed on this aspect of Pasteur's character and suggested that he may have tailored his scientific pronouncements to political pressures because (as will be noted below) Lawson Tait thought there were weaknesses in Pasteur's teaching. It is by no means irrelevant to the matter that Tait does seem to have studied Pouchet's works much more deeply than did most of his scientific or medical contemporaries.

Despite all the evidence accumulated by Pasteur and the support generated by the successful application of his theories in Lister's work, many remained convinced of the doctrine of spontaneous generation as far as micro-organisms were concerned. Henry Bastian (1837-1915), a physician whose life work was divided between neurology and bacteriology, in 1867 contradicted some of Pasteur's crucial results and so prolonged the controversy. Pasteur eventually refuted Bastian's work by further experiments (and, incidentally, in doing so perfected sterilisation methods by introducing the autoclave and the sterilisation of materials by steam under pressure). Despite this defeat Bastian went on until the end of his days preaching the gospel of spontaneous generation in numerous papers and in repeated editions of his book *The Origin of Life.*

We may now see how Lawson Tait was influenced by all these developments and how he applied them to his surgical thinking. It must be confessed that at times his ideas were rather confused and their practical application illogical. The influence of those who taught him as a student in Edinburgh remained strong all his life. In 1898, in one of his last papers attacking Listerism, he ends by asserting that "if we had watched Syme more closely and had listened to Simpson with ear other than that of the adder, closed and deaf, we had not needed this fight." This was an over-simplification of his lifelong creed but it emphasises that basically he always believed that absolute cleanliness in surgical technique and an unpolluted environment (the first stressed by Syme and the second by Simpson) were more important in the eradication of sepsis than was Lister's doctrine. He had soon become aware also of Thomas Keith's remarkable success in ovariotomy achieved without any antiseptic precautions.

It is from a lecture which Tait delivered in Birmingham in 1887 that we learn something of his early studies and the evolution of his ideas.[34] He recalled how while he was in Wakefield he had read (in 1868) Pouchet's *L'Origine de la Vie* and that it had remained "a landmark in his life." He continued, "I now know that many of his conclusions were incomplete and many of his observations inaccurate by reason of his faulty apparatus, but his book kept me out of the errors of the school of Pasteur, and freed me from the dreams of Lister. . . ."

Tait went on to describe how he had studied all the papers of Pasteur, Tyndall and Bastian and that in his interpretation of these writers he was "tinctured by the strongest belief in the faith of Darwin." He did not consider that anyone who accepted Darwin's teaching could possibly believe in Listerism. His reasoning on this point is rather unclear, but it appears that certain bacteriological work in the early seventies—for example, Büchner's demonstration that by successive cultures he had changed the virulent anthrax bacillus to a harmless organism — was in his (Tait's) view a complete contradiction of Darwin's theory. In accepting Darwinism Tait had to admit that the theory of spontaneous generation was quite unacceptable and that Pouchet and Bastian were wrong. This might make it appear that Tait should have progressed rapidly to the germ theory of disease, but he did not do so. Although he accepted the argument that if a sterilised fluid like beef tea was placed in a hermetically sealed vessel it would remain fresh, because no microorganisms could come in contact with it, and recognised also that carefully filtered air would not cause infection of a culture medium, he was not prepared to go along with Lister and apply such observations to wound management. Instead, he became involved in a rather woolly exposition. Of the theories of Pasteur and Lister he affirmed that "they did not give prominence to other facts." He philosophised about "vital power" or a "life-force". From a confused series of general observations he tried to show that the key to the understanding of wound infection lay in making a distinction between dead and living tissue. He made his case by somewhat shaky analogies. For instance, he said that "there is not a henwife in the kingdom that does not know that fertilised hen's eggs stay fresh for a long time in an incubator while non-fertilised eggs go putrid in a short time."[35] He attributed this to the presence in the fertilised egg of a "very minute mass of tissue which when living seems to possess the most extraordinary powers not only of resisting decomposition itself but of preserving from decomposition the non-organised mass of albumen with which it is associated." Here was his mysterious life-force at work ; indeed, "if the scientific workers had known as much as the henwife they would have known that to apply the conclusions derived from beef tea in the flasks of the chemist's laboratory to the phenomena of living tissue is nonsense."

Tait was emphasising something very important – namely, that bacterial action was more likely to occur in the presence of dead tissue than in living tissue. He was more interested in the soil than in the seed: "the germs are the same – it is the vital condition of the nidus which changes." This was an important principle to express but it is difficult to see what it had to do with rejecting the antiseptic methods of Lister.

By now Tait was confessing that he could not keep up with all the new theories and discoveries of the bacteriologists. As many of the more important new ideas came from Germans he was even less disposed to listen. He had a poor opinion of German scientists: "the German medical mind is essentially different from that of the Briton. . . . Nothing pleases it as much as metaphysical speculation whilst we, on the contrary, are eminently pragmatic."

This paper, presumably a challenge to Lister, was rather a failure. It was confused, illogical and ill-supported by exact observation or experiment. In a subsequent paper in 1891 Tait stated:[36]

> In conclusion let me again say that as the wrecks of the cellular pathology remain to us valuable contributions towards the solutions of the mysteries of disease: as the construction by Bennet of a scheme of molecular pathology did much to help us, so has the germ theory rendered us a great service. But as a final answer it is insufficient and its wholesale and reckless application is alike mischievous and misleading.

To the end of his life Tait went on presenting obscure statements: "Sepsis was related to some potent influence capable of being carried from one patient to another, nobody knowing how. . . . certain symptoms with pyrexia appear, nobody knowing why." His ideas about a mysterious life-force or vitality were summarised in three sentences:

> The germs of putrefaction exist, with restrained potentiality, in all living creatures.
> That the restraining influence is what we call, for want of a better term, the vital force.
> That when the restraining influence has been upset by what we call disease, lowered vitality etc. the germs are let loose to work their evil ways.

Such hypotheses were not likely to convince anyone, least of all Lister. As Tait admitted that he had not time to follow the advances in bacteriology, such as those presented by Koch, his ideas were even less likely to be taken seriously. One comment on a paper by Tait in 1881 reads, "We do not think this paper will materially obstruct the progress of the greatest reform in wound treatment of the present day."

While the flow of criticism from Tait continued for some 30 years he did give occasional, if grudging, acknowledgment of Lister's contributions to surgery. There were few direct confrontations and it is doubtful if the two men met very often. There was one particular passage of arms between them in 1890. In that year Lister addressed the International Medical Congress in Berlin.[37] He revealed that he (in contrast to Tait) had followed closely the expansion of bacteriology and, in particular, that he had met Koch and discussed with him problems relevant to surgical practice. He had studied the new theory of Metchnicoff of the action of the white cells of the blood (phagocytes) in devouring bacteria. In this phenomenon Lister saw the explanation of a "potent force" which living tissue seemed to exert in checking bacterial proliferation in a wound. Lister also referred to Tait's insistence that abdominal operations were successful without antiseptic techniques. Lister admitted his own lack of experience in this field of surgery but gave explanations for Tait's good results. He confessed that he had now abandoned the spray, saying, "I feel ashamed that I should have ever recommended it for destroying the microbes of the air." This admission showed both his humility and his greatness, for he had for long believed that the spray was an important part of his technique, perhaps the most important. He had now transferred his allegiance from carbolic acid to cyanide of zinc or mercury as an antiseptic agent. There was no reference to the new school of "aseptic" surgery which was now being established; that Lister had no objection to the term "aseptic" is explained by the fact that he saw in this conception only a slight variation of his own antiseptic principles.

Tait had a less important audience for a reply, which he made in a paper entitled "An address on the present aspect of antiseptic surgery" delivered to the East Anglian Branch of the British Medical Association at Cromer.[38] He started with a long and (perhaps to his audience) a rather wearisome review of early ideas of inflammation from Stahl's phlogiston theory, through Lavoisier's and Priestley's researches on oxygen—which cancelled out the phlogiston theory—and finally to Lister's principles. The latter he described as "not a theory at all but an absolute and ludicrous logical error." He considered Darwin to be one of the few scientists able to construct a working hypothesis and then find a series of facts to fit it. (Tait was not very good at this exercise himself!) He did not rate Koch's discoveries in bacteriology very highly and thought little of Metchnicoff's phagocyte theory except as an extension of a concept which had long since been revealed to Tait as a student, for he recalled how the Professor of Natural History in Edinburgh demonstrated the "all-devouring amoeba." But the matter which offended was Lister's reference to Tait's experience of ovariotomy. He insisted that by this Lister had been given an absolute refutation of the antiseptic system but that he had taken no notice of this evidence. The paper ended in a challenge to Lister to produce adequate statistics of his results, a challenge which others such as Savory had offered and for which there was a certain amount of justification.

If Tait's vague theoretical objections weakened his case, he perhaps had already fallen into a greater error when he launched an attack in 1882. At the annual meeting of the British Medical Association in Worcester he read a paper to the Surgical Section entitled "One Hundred Consecutive Cases of Ovariotomy performed without any of the Listerian Details".[39] This was the theme of repeated attempts to overthrow Lister's doctrines and it is clear that he backed the wrong horse! There were only three deaths in this series, a remarkable success which he ascribed to several factors—his abandonment of Wells' clamp technique, the adoption of Keith's method of cleansing the abdominal cavity, the establishment of scrupulous hospital discipline and hygiene, but most of all the complete discard "of the use of carbolic acid or any other antiseptic system." He had previously produced some rather confused statistics of the results of ovariotomy with and without antiseptic precautions, but this paper announced his irrevocable abandonment of Listerism.

Tait's exceptional success in abdominal surgery could not be used as a convincing argument against the antiseptic system. Lister had applied his methods especially in the management of compound fractures and acute abscesses. He had from the first recognised certain limitations as far as abdominal operations were concerned. Although he seldom performed such procedures himself he had sent his cases of ovarian cysts for many years to Keith, the foremost ovariotomist in Scotland, and he had watched closely the evolution of this operation. In 1881 Lister set forth his firm view on this subject:[40]

> Ovariotomy indeed has sometimes been spoken of as a touchstone of the efficacy of the antiseptic treatment. . . . Such, however, has never been my own view. Mr. Spencer Wells and Dr. Thos. Keith achieved results which astonished the world before antiseptic treatmen was thought of: and when Dr. Keith expressed to me an intention of performing ovariotomy antiseptically I strongly dissuaded him from his purpose. I knew his already brilliant success: I felt that our spray apparatus was as yet inadequate for the production of a cloud sufficiently large to cover the whole field of operation and sufficiently fine to avoid needless irritation. . . . It seemed to me in any case of ovariotomy performed without antiseptic measures there was a contest between effusion from the wounded surfaces and absorption by the uninjured peritoneum. If absorption kept pace with effusion there was no time for putrefactive fermentation to take place . . . but if absorption lagged behind and effusion predominated the serum accumulated in the abdominal cavity and, putrefying, gave rise to septicaemia. Now supposing an antiseptic like carbolic acid to be employed in the operation, the peritoneal surfaces, as well as those of the wound would be more or less irritated by it and in proportion to this irritation would effusion be increased and absorbing power enfeebled. . . and if in spite of the antiseptic means active septic matter had been introduced putrefaction and septicaemia would be the natural result.
>
> But how, it may naturally be asked, can the success of ovariotomy performed without the use of antiseptic means be reconciled with the truth of the antiseptic principle? The answer is, I believe, to be found in certain peculiarities of the abdominal cavity . . . . The plasma from the cut surface is poured into a large cavity lined with a serous membrane disposed to absorb it as fast as it is effused. A further peculiarity in favour of abdominal wounds is due to the high vital power of the peritoneum.

The last rather vague sentence should have appealed to Tait. Lister was stating a fact already known to many surgeons such as Keith and Spencer Wells and accepted with gratitude by the abdominal surgeon today, that the peritoneum has a remarkable natural power to cope with trauma and infection. Lister knew very well that this exceptional absorptive power of the peritoneum might be dangerous if carbolic acid from the spray or other sources was introduced into the abdominal cavity in quantity, for it would readily poison the patient by absorption into the bloodstream. On several occasions Tait had written of severe toxic effects associated with the excessive use of the spray in abdominal operations, but he did not seem to have appreciated the fact that Lister had warned of this danger.

Lister's clear exposition was the answer to the main argument which Tait brought against the antiseptic method. Tait was obstinate and refused to accept defeat. He did insist that he had tried the method for compound fractures and more recently for breast operations, but it must be accepted that now most of his work was in the abdomen. He tried to reinforce his argument when his many large series of abdominal sections were published in succeeding years. Lister largely ignored all these attacks; he rightly felt that he had said the last word and that Tait could be calmly and politely ignored.

It is worth noting that Thomas Keith, who had been so successful in his ovariotomy results before adopting Listerian methods, discarded these quickly and returned to simple aseptic methods, thus giving some support to Tait. In 1885 Keith gave an account of his recent experience with hysterectomy "with remarks on the Carbolic Acid Spray in abdominal surgery."[41]

> The antiseptic principle can be carried out by simpler means. . . for myself I have almost gone back to the boiled water and soda of twenty years ago. It is unfortunately a sad fact that, ever since surgery began, the great evil was done by the surgeon himself. It was he, willing and tender, through unclean hand that carried most of the poison into the wound. It is to this that Lister has put a stop. With a proper antiseptic a surgeon is now made to be clean in spite of himself, is compelled to have safe sponges, safe ligatures, clean instruments and above all clean fingers. If we be careful enough—and few are careful enough, we may do all this, as Mr. Lawson Tait does with boiled water and soda. Some sound precautions are essential; beyond these with ordinary care we need not disturb ourselves much as to what is in the air. Yet it was a pleasant doctrine to believe, to put the blame of a bad result. . . . upon something indefinite, something in the air. . . .

Keith was primarily giving his reasons for discarding the spray but he was showing also that he, having grasped the essentials of Lister's theory, could nevertheless depart from the antiseptic to an aseptic method.

In summary, Tait did not deny that wound infection was associated in some way with micro-organisms, but he was not convinced that these caused the phenomena of wound infection. He insisted that it was an error to apply the experimental work on putrefaction to the phenomena of disease in living tissues. As has been shown, he concentrated instead on the idea that the soil was more important than the seed—how otherwise, he argued, was there not a fatal result every time an individual pricked his skin? Gradually he discarded in his own practice most of the details of the antiseptic technique. He was right in discarding the spray, for as Lister himself was eventually to admit, it was ineffective as well as a source of great discomfort to the operator and his staff and when used in operations of the abdomen it was a dangerous source of irritation and toxicity. He soon discarded carbolic acid solutions in the preparation of the skin before an operation, for both the sterilisation of his instruments as well as for use as an antiseptic material in his dressings. He was glad to give up the preparation of his hands by immersion in carbolic acid solutions which irritated and coarsened the skin (rubber gloves were not devised until 1894 and there is no record that Tait or Lister ever used them).

How then did Tait achieve such great success after discarding all Lister's methods by which the latter had brought about such a remarkable improvement in the control of serious sepsis? The answer lies partly in the fact that when he moved to Birmingham Tait did not operate in conditions so grossly septic as those of the Glasgow Royal Infirmary and so dangerous in most large hospitals in Great Britain. He worked instead in small hospitals where he ensured a standard of cleanliness far above those of most large establishments. He maintained a discipline over his nursing staff far more effectively than most of his contemporaries. It is true that the technique he evolved was in the main applied to abdominal surgery but there *was* a large wound liable to be infected at operation or at repeated dressing, however remarkable were the powers of the peritoneum to resist infection.

The details of Tait's technique were as follows. He substituted for Lister's application of a carbolic acid solution to the skin of the operative site a simple but thorough cleansing with soap and water (but if the patient "was a poor dirty creature" he did use turpentine!). Tait prepared his hands by careful toilet with soap and hot water and a nail brush; Lister used a strong lotion of carbolic acid. Lister took off his jacket and pinned an unsterilised towel to his waistcoat; Tait donned a large, clean mackintosh apron. During an operation Lister worked with a constant supply of towels soaked in carbolic around the operation field and as long as he used the spray he applied it continually to the wound, to the instruments and to his hands. Tait washed his hands in warm water from time to time throughout the operation but used no antiseptic fluids. Marine sponges were in popular use for mopping up blood or other fluids and were perhaps the most dangerous source of all infections, for they were supplied in a dirty condition and were almost impossible to clean thoroughly because of their porous nature. Tait was meticulous in the care of his sponges, treating them with a solution of washing soda or ammonia; sometimes (rather inconsistently) he soaked them in carbolic acid solution for a week and finally washed them out thoroughly with boiled water immediately before use. It was a long time before the marine sponge was discarded, whether it was treated with carbolic (as by Lister) or by Tait's method. In any case, it must always have been a dangerous source of infection, particularly since the sponges were used again and again! Instead of carbolised catgut, which Lister prepared for himself in the most meticulous way, Tait used silk sterilised by boiling. Finally, Tait did not see the necessity for antiseptic dressings in the post-operative period but followed Gamgee's system of dry wool dressings.

Tait's ideas about surgical technique are summarised in a lecture he gave in Birmingham in 1891:[42]

> We who are opposed to the antiseptic doctrines and the antiseptic practices argued that the germs were harmless if dead and dying material on which they may feed were removed from the wound. The washing out of the abdomen, therefore, for the removal of all clots, dirt and debris and the free use of the drainage tube, formed the complementary practice to essential cleanliness and paved the way to our enormous advances in abdominal surgery. I venture to predict that four or five years hence the use of the term "antiseptics" will be dropped and we shall hear no more of this strange phase of surgical eccentricity.

From practical experience Tait developed something very close to aseptic surgery, for he tried to achieve absolute cleanliness, using sterile materials as much as he could. There was a more difficult problem in traumatic surgery when wounds were already infected, and it must be admitted that he did not emphasise the need to use antiseptics in such cases; in any event, this ceased to be an important matter in his later surgical career. He did, however, operate frequently on the septic abdomen and it was in this kind of surgery that he worked to combat infection by simple irrigation of the abdominal cavity, at first with ordinary tap water. He delighted in boasting that although the Birmingham city analyst had found at least 30 varieties of micro-organisms in the water supply these never caused trouble. Perhaps it was just as well that he soon changed to boiled water!

If the theorics on which he based his practice were confused, his results improved from year to year as far as abdominal surgery was concerned and justified his methods. Perhaps most important of all was his appreciation of the fact that in septic cases he must remove blood-clot and other debris which otherwise would provide a nidus for infection. He was a strong advocate of drainage for septic conditions. He had learnt from Simpson the need to avoid unnecessary trauma to wounds, to remove damaged tissue and to ligate vessels neatly in order to avoid the retention in a cavity of large stumps of dead tissue.

Most writers ascribe to German surgeons such as Von Bergmann the introduction of the aseptic system of surgery—that is, an operative technique for clean or elective surgery almost completely without the use of any antiseptic methods. There is some evidence that, in abdoinal surgery at least, Tait's technique was by 1880 more aseptic than that of any of the Germans. In 1892 McKay visited Von Bergmann and found that he was still soaking his instruments in carbolic acid and using antiseptics to prepare his sponges. It is almost impossible and perhaps unimportant to determine priority as far as aseptic surgery is concerned. The evolution from antiseptic to aseptic surgery was a gradual process and surgeons in many different countries contributed to this advance. The trasition was perhaps more rapid in Germany where Lister's teaching was generally taken up more urgently than in Great Britain or America. In the particular field of abdominal surgery Lawson Tait and Thomas Keith may be singled out, however, as pioneers in their development of aseptic techniques. The one (Tait) almost completely and obstinately refused to admit that Lister had shown the way to this practice; the other (Keith) recognised that Lister's principles could be readily accommodated to the idea of aseptic surgery.

Quarrels over the antiseptic system were often petty and pointless, and it could be said that Tait was bigoted and unscientific in the way he waged his battle with Lister. However, the argument did have beneficial results—it hastened the transition from the elaborate (and sometimes unnecessary) and often tedious antiseptic technique to the simpler aseptic method. In clean or elective surgery the modern surgeon comes closer in his methods to Tait than to Lister, but this cannot take away from Lister his achievement in correcting the appalling situation of about 1865 and in establishing surgery as a science as well as an art.

CHAPTER VII

Disciple of Charles Darwin

In 1885 Lawson Tait recalled, "in my short life nothing has given me more satisfaction than my association with Charles Darwin, first as a fervent disciple, and afterwards as a humble follower and friend." As a student, perhaps as early as 1860, he had read the *Origin of Species.* We have recorded how he made the new theories the subject of his presidential address to a student society, very likely incurring the wrath of his teachers. If he was not present at Thomas Huxley's lectures in Edinburgh in January 1862 on "Man's place in Nature" he must at least have been aware of the storm created by this exposition of Darwinism.[1]

When Tait moved to Wakefield he developed further his interest in evolution; he read all he could lay hands on, he debated the question in the local societies and in 1869 he wrote his article on Natural Selection for the *Dublin Quarterly Journal of Medicine.* This controversial paper was a matter of no small pride to Tait when Darwin referred to it in his first edition of the *Descent of Man.* Tait (and other critics) made the point that the law of natural selection might operate adversely in civilised communities. Darwin accepted and developed this view, writing that "excepting in the case of man himself, hardly anyone is so ignorant as to allow his worst animals to breed."[2]

Tait established close contacts with Darwin, and it is possible to trace from surviving letters the extent of their collaboration. The correspondence reveals some unexpected facets of Tait's character and of his interests outside surgery. That even as a student he should have grasped so positively the importance of Darwin's contribution to biology is noteworthy; that as a busy surgeon he should have become so deeply involved in this scientific controversy is remarkable. In the early sixties there were not many who recognised that Darwin's theory of evolution was the most important general advance ever made in the field of biology. Those few medically qualified men who were early to grasp the significance of Darwin's work (and its possible application to medicine) were mostly botanists, zoologists and the like. Only a handful of practising surgeons or physicians, in the early years, took note of Darwin's work and were aware of its relevance to medical science. Amongst the few, James Paget (1814-1899) was the most closely involved with Darwin and provided him with much useful detail of human anatomy and pathology. Paget's numerous letters to Darwin were described by his son as "those of a disciple to a master: the one desire is to collect facts and make observations for him." Paget wrote to Darwin in 1869:[3]

> I thank you with all my heart for sending me your book (the variation of animals and plants under domestication.) I shall refresh and teach myself with it. . . . I expect to be made even more than I am now ashamed of my ignorance (and I fear of my profession too) on the influence of inheritance on the variations and mixtures of diseases. But I hope that my deeper shame may be the beginning of deeper knowledge.

Paget had good reason to comment on the lack of interest of his profession. The *Lancet* made no reference to Darwin in the five years following the publication of the *Origin. The British Medical Journal* first noticed Darwin in 1861, but only by the reproduction of some light verse from *Blackwood's Magazine.*[4]

> From reptiles and fishes we ascend,
> And quadrupeds next their dimensions extend,
> Till we rise up to monkeys and men—where we end.

Perhaps this was just about as much as the average doctor could be expected to assimilate and accounts for the fact that the importance to medicine of Darwin's work was for long unappreciated.

William Turner (1832-1914) had gone to Edinburgh, after working with Paget in London, to be a Demonstrator in Anatomy under Professor Goodsir. Turner became Professor in 1867. Unlike Goodsir, he was prepared to go a long way towards accepting Darwin's theories. Like Paget, Turner corresponded frequently with Darwin and supplied him with details of anatomy and, on occasion, with criticisms and corrections of his writings.[5]

In July 1871 we found the young Tait intervening in the great controversy by contributing a short letter to *Nature.* The first letter between Darwin and Tait which can be traced is an acknowledgement by Darwin of information which had been sent to him on a matter of anatomical interest: (b)

Oct. 8 1871

Dear Sir,

I do not know anything about a supracondyloid process in the humerus yet I have a vague remembrance of having heard of it.

But my knowledge of anatomy is quite insufficient to be trusted. If you publish on this subject I shd. be grateful for a copy of your paper.

Dear Sir, Yours very faithfully

Ch. Darwin.

Darwin's comment was a little surprising, for he had just published *The Descent of Man,* in which he supported his views on evolution by reference to certain rudimentary or vestigial structures found in the human, such as the appendix and the branchial or gill clefts in the neck. He also drew attention to the supracondyloid foramen, a bony passage in the lower end of the humerus through which a major artery and nerve are transmitted in the ape and an arrangement seen in the human as an incomplete bony channel. Darwin had, in addition, written to William Turner in March 1871 thanking him for correcting certain errors he had made in describing this developmental condition.

There is no record of a subsequent paper by Tait on this subject. It is clear, however, that Tait had now begun to supply Darwin with information which might be useful to him, just as Paget and Turner were doing.

In 1873 Tait published a "Note on a poly-dactylus cat from Cookham Dean" in the journal *Nature.* Darwin, in his first edition of the *Origin of Species*, had stated that cats with blue eyes were invariably deaf. In a later edition he corrected this statement and acknowledged that Tait had convinced him that deafness occurred in white cats of the male sex, irrespective of eye colour. Tait described one of his own pet cats, "Pudge", a deaf white male, with one blue and one yellow eye and with supernumerary digits. In 1884 he had to report, however, that he had observed deafness in white female cats, although he still believed the association was more common in males. He took the trouble to have the ears of a deaf female cat examined and reported that a congenital gap was found in the tympanic membrane.

Before 1875 communications between the two men were probably sporadic, but meanwhile Tait was now boldly preaching the doctrines of Darwin in Birmingham to local societies and to the enthusiastic ladies who attended his biology class. This particular activity scandalised some of his colleagues and some local churchmen. In 1875 Tait began to bombard Darwin with questions and with his own ideas. Darwin replied promptly and with great courtesy to almost all these letters despite the fact that he was usually in the throes of research, writing, or reading proof and was often extremely exhausted. In 1875 Tait began to review Darwin's works for the *Spectator*, which he continued to do for several years.

In all we have traced a total of twenty-nine letters from Tait to Darwin and twenty-one from Darwin to Tait in the years 1875 and 1876. It can be inferred that many others passed between them. In March 1875 Tait gives Darwin an account of his cat and some of his theories concerning the functions of tails: (a)

March 12 (1875)

Dear Sir,

I have had previous occasion to correspond with you on subjects bearing on evolution, and there is one more little matter in which I would like your opinion. As one of your disciples it has been my object to try the doctrine of evolution by survival of fitness at every possible point and amongst other things I have speculated on the origin of tails.

For every tail I got a satisfactory reason save for the bushy tail of such animals as the civet cat, some dogs, wolf etc. That variety long puzzled me until the accidental observation of a favourite white cat, who is perfectly deaf, solved the riddle to me.

On him I can perform experiments by reason of his deafness, without arousing his suspicion and I find that he uses his tail as a respirator to keep up his temperature. I catch him asleep before a German stove, lying at full length on his side with tail and limbs stretched out to enjoy the full heat. Then I intercept the heat by a screen and without waking he gradually coils himself up so as to cover as much surface as possible to save loss of heat. Then when I drive a current of cold air on him from a pair of bellows he twines his tail round him and buries his nose completely in the fur between it and the thigh, thereby establishing a natural respirator which must conserve his temperature to a very remarked extent. Birds do the same thing when they bury their noses in their wings. I cannot find a bushy tailed animal which cannot curl itself up. If I could any theory would be spoilt. I mentioned this to my friend Professor Haughton of Dublin a few days ago when on a visit to him and on a very cold morning we started round the Zoological Gardens to examine for the point. We found the civet cat and others coiled up and their noses covered with their fur. I do not know whether the observation is an original one or not, but it is at any rate interesting.

I purpose communicating a short note on it to the Birmingham Natural History Society and previous to that I should like to know your opinion of my theory.

Yours faithfully

Lawson Tait.

Five days later there was another letter in which Tait switched to a different topic, the growth of tumours of the ovary. (a)

March 17 (1875)

Dear Sir,

Another matter I should like to draw your attention to. I send by this post a short essay which I wrote a few months ago and I should like you to read pp. 58-63.

I think there is a pathological interest in the curious tumours mentioned there which bears on evolution.

The more I think over some of the problems of pathology the more I lean towards the view that their solution will be aided by regarding them from a Darwinian point of view.

When you have read the passage referred to and have leisure I should be much gratified by having your opinion about it.

Yours truly

Lawson Tait.

Next day there followed another letter on tails with the description of some experiments. (a)

March 18 (1875)

Dear Sir,

Thanks for your kind note. I shall send you a copy of my little paper.

I am keeping a number of white mice to try to unravel the use of the peculiar tail of mice and rats but I am completely beaten.

My view does not preclude any other modification or use of the tail: but it seems to me to be important as illustrating how correlation of growth (that is thick fur lending to a bushy tail) will bring out a new circumstance favourable to survival and therefore lead to a total alteration of some important habits—as the curling up of these animals when going to sleep.

Yours faithfully

Lawson Tait.

Tait eventually published some of his observations on tails in *Nature* in 1879. The paper which he sent to Darwin was, of course, his Hastings Essay on ovarian disease. Darwin was particularly interested in the developmental tumours which were described and he wrote a letter which must have given great pleasure to Tait. (c)

March 20 (1875)

Dear Sir,

I have read with *much* interest that part of your essay which you point out and I hope hereafter to read the whole. I have not knowledge enough to form an opinion of any value on your view. But the facts which you give about these tumours, such as the enclosed teeth etc. (tho' I had never heard of the more wonderful cases you refer to) seem to me highly favourable to some such notion as that of pangenesis: for they indicate that there must be independent germs for each part. . . .

Dear Sir

Yours faithfully

Ch. Darwin

For some years Darwin had been developing his theory of pangenesis. He had discussed it in his book *The Variation of Plants and Animals under Domestication,* published in 1868. In 1875 Darwin rewrote his concept of this process, a somewhat obscure attempt to deal with genetic problems which could not be explained by the theory of evolution. He believed that all fully differentiated tissues were represented in the germ cells by "gemmules" or "buds" which determined the growth of specific cells. Tait's descriptions of ovarian tumours containing recognisable hair, teeth or other tissues gave Darwin some support for his idea of pangenesis. On his part Tait saw possibilities in the acceptance of this theory in relation to tumour formation. He produced, however, an alternative theory of "hypererchesis". This too was a rather obscure idea that tissue growth was determined by the action of "origin-buds" in the ovary.[6]

Perhaps encouraged by this cordial reply Tait now sought a meeting with Darwin. In 1842 he had moved from London to Down, near Orpington in Kent, to seek seclusion and to nurse his energies by limiting his writing and other work to a few hours each day. He was subject to depressive attacks with excessive fatigue as a prominent symptom. It is difficult to accept the idea that there was any physical basis for his symptoms. Darwin wrote to Alfred Wallace in 1862: "My health is, and always will be, very poor: I am that miserable animal a regular valetudinarian." Some of his prolonged illnesses followed the strain of reading the proofs of his books. In the Spring of 1875 he was very tired after completing the second edition of *The Variation of Plants and Animals under Domestication* and his monograph on the insectivorous plants was then in preparation. At the end of March he was also rather exhausted by the frequent sittings he had to give to the artist Ouless, who did produce an exceptionally good portrait. (Darwin, however, observed "I look a very venerable, acute melancholy, old dog.") (c)

March 25 1875

Dear Sir,

I am much obliged by your kind note. I should be very glad to make your personal acquaintance and no introduction was in the least necessary. I fear however that we cannot meet just at present. I have long been much out of health, and lately I have been working very hard and am quite knocked up: at the best of times I cannot converse with any one for more than half an hour or so; and at present I should be incapable even of this much exertion. Therefore I beg you to propose some future Sunday. But I am going on the 31st or 1st for a week to my brother's house 6, Queen Anne St., Cavendish Square, for complete rest and expect that two or three days will set me up. Down is rather an awkward place to reach, and if it would suit you better to come to London on the 4th or on one of the few succeeding days I should have great pleasure in seeing you. I would suggest your coming to luncheon and then we could have some talk afterwards. But in this case please to inform me so that I may keep myself fresh.

My dear Sir

Yours very faithfully

Ch. Darwin

Tait tactfully turned down the suggestion to meet in London and suggested that he should come to Down early in April. (a)

March 27 (1875)

Dear Sir,

It would not be fair in me to intrude when you are at rest in London, so that I would rather visit you after your return to Down, say on the 11th, 18th or 25th.

For years I have been working at details of the great scheme you have sketched out and of course the more I get into it, the more vast and intricate it becomes yet the more universally applicable seem the laws.

As I am not hampered by worldly exigencies, I do not devote myself to the drudgery of medical life and therefore have time for science. I am at present preparing a paper for the Royal Society on the Umbilical cord and some of the conclusions to which I am led have so startled me that I merely hint at them in this preliminary note (to the R.S.). Thus the spiral form of the cord, which has been thought by us a mere anatomical curiosity seems to me to bear strongly on the evidence of the descent of man and here I want your advice and assistance. It has further led me to a hypothesis for the spiral growth of plants—and therefore the spiral growth of everything, which I wish to submit to your criticism.

I shall endeavour not to weary you.

Please do not answer this note save to fix one of these Sundays or some [other day] still later on, at Down.

Yours faithfully
Lawson Tait.

Both Tait's comment about "worldly exigencies" and his suggestion that he had plenty of spare time for scientific study are a little surprising. By now he was heavily committed to his practice and involved in an increasing number of activities. Perhaps he feared that Darwin might not take a full-time surgeon seriously as a fellow scientist! The paper on the umbilical cord referred to in this letter was communicated on Tait's behalf to the Royal Society by William Savory F.R.S. later in the year. Darwin may well have been interested in this study of the microscopic structure of the cord and in the reasons which Tait advanced for the spiral arrangement of its vessels.[7]

The visit took place on Sunday April the 18th. Tait arrived early in the morning at Orpington Station and was probably met by Darwin's coachman. He had been told that Thomas Huxley would be there and this was an added attraction. Breakfast was probably taken with Mrs. Darwin and those of the family who were at home; Darwin usually took his breakfast alone. Perhaps Tait was given an hour's discussion after breakfast and then the great man would have retired to his study. At midday a visitor might have had the privilege of strolling and talking with Darwin through the grounds of Down by the Sand Walk. Lunch was a family meal and after another short discussion Darwin would most likely have retired to rest again.[8]

Visitors were frequent to Down but not all of them saw much of Darwin. He did, however, go out of his way to entertain young and enthusiastic scientists who had still to make their name. For Tait the visit proved to be one of the most important events of his life and he often recalled it. It may be presumed that discussion ranged over a wide variety of subjects. There may have been reference to Darwin's early days in Edinburgh as a student but the theory of evolution must have predominated. There was certainly discussion about insectivorous plants and the delicate matter of Tait's possible election to the Royal Society was raised. Shortly after the meeting Darwin wrote to Tait: (c)

April 29 (1875)

My Dear Sir,

Prof. Dyer says it would take much time to look up all the references about Nepenthe. . . .

With respect to your candidature for R. Soc., I of course know nothing, but I believe the Council judge as well as they can (and take infinite pains) just what he has actually published, but are influenced somewhat by the estimation in which he is held, and considerably by the length of time during which he has been a candidate.

Yours vy. faithfully

Ch. Darwin.

Darwin had started to write his book on insectivorous plants in 1874.[9] He finished it in March and it was published in July 1875. It seems that Tait became intensely interested in this botanical subject about the time of his visit to Darwin. There were now frequent letters about this new topic. (a)

June 2 (1875)

My Dear Sir,

Dr. Burdon Sanderson's paper on the leaf currents in Dionoea has set me observing the insectivorous plants, and I wait longingly for your book, that I may see more wonders.

But some of my independent observations are most curious and one which mere accident has revealed is so startling that I hasten to send it to you, even at the risk of it being already known to you.

This afternoon I was hurriedly summoned from my plants and I left a Drosera uncovered in a hot drawing room exposed to a full glare of sunshine. When I came back in a few hours it seemed drained, the leaf stalks being much shrunken. Its traps were all open, so I tried to see if its nervous system was dead.

I found that irritation of a nerve fibre (and we must I think give them that name) of one side of the traps caused incurvation of the fingers and closure of the flap on the opposite side only!

That is reflex action and as we find reflex action of the most remarked in certain forms of disease and injury which induce paralysis, it seems to me it occurs in this plant.

For instance, in health, tickling the inside of the thigh does not induce elevation of the testicle by contraction of the cremaster muscle save in the infant but after fracture of the spine it nearly always does. My poor dionoea therefore was paralysed.

From what I have seen I am sure we shall find still greater reason to allow a nervous system for these plants.

I am watching a lot of my mice from whom I removed the tails at birth, and I am coming to the conclusion that the essential use of the tail is as a recording organ, that is they record in their memories the corners they turn and the height of the holes they pass through by touching them with their tails. Is not this queer?

With best regards to Mrs. Darwin and with tender recollection of my visit to Down. I remain

Yours ever

Lawson Tait.

We may wonder if Tait realised that Darwin had been studying the insectivorous plants since 1860 and had done meticulous experiments on the Sundew (Drosera) to determine the functions of its tentacles and the mode of digesting its prey. He had already considered the possibility of a nervous mechanism to account for the extreme sensitivity of the plant. In 1874 he had analysed the secretions of Drosera and found an acid of the acetic series and a ferment which he thought was analogous to "pepsine". Tait's rather amateurish observations could not have been new to Darwin but he replied on June 4th indicating that he had been much interested, giving hints on how to conduct further experiments and advancing his own theories of nervous action. Darwin was perhaps more interested in the progress of Tait's experiments on mice and remarked that "If you make out about the tails of mice it will be a beautiful discovery." Tait answered the very next day. (a)

June 5 (1875)

My Dear Sir,

I am very grateful for your letter. The dodge of making incisions is new to me and I shall try it.

I purpose giving a lecture on "Insect-Eating plants" to our local Natural History Society on the 15th and if it should meet with approval I shall publish it. May I dedicate it to you? Silence will give consent. . . .

If I can ever at any time relieve you of any drudgery in correcting proof, pray let me know. My wife does all mine and she is the sharpest hand at it I have ever met with. She will be delighted to ease the labour of one whose writings she knows so well.

I am now at liberty to pursue the tail question, as I have just delivered my Magnum Opus to the Royal Society in the hope of its leading to my admission to that sanctum, the FRS being my greatest ambition. The paper is on the umbilical cord and I think that I shall yet be able to draw upon it a great illustration of evolution. It will be read on the 17th.

Yours faithfully

Lawson Tait.

Darwin wrote to thank Mrs. Tait for her offer to help with his proofs but he feared that it was indispensable for him to correct his own writings. He suggested that Tait should make some sections of mice tails ("if you are accustomed to such histological work"); He thought that hairs on the mouse's tail might have sensitive nerves, as had been reported in the hairs on the ears of some animals. On June 12 Tait dashed off two letters. In both he reported more experimental work. (a)

June 12. (1875)

My Dear Sir,

Another point that may interest you. The glands of Drosera dichotoma (Australian) are constantly covered with a viscid secretion, its action being exactly that of the D. Rotundofolia.

I gathered a lot of the fluid and by Brücke's method I have been able to separate a nitrogenous matter with a very close resemblance to pepsin.

It is not pepsin but I propose meantime to call it droserin. If you would like the details of my experiments and the process I shall be glad to send them. It has a curious action on milk, amongst other things, resembling but not identical with rennet. I suppose you know that old Gerrard says that Dr. rot. was very much used in Cheshire in his days for rennet.

I have just had a summons and am just off to Shrewsbury.

Yours faithfully

Lawson Tait.

[P.S.] Please don't trouble to write an answer to this more than a post card to say if you would like the particulars.

June 12 (1875)

My Dear Sir,

Your letter has just arrived after the posting of my first. I am really ashamed that you should take up so much of your time in answering my letters. My only excuse in troubling you at all is that younger workers reap in the great field you have sown.

Many thanks for the references. I shall hunt them up.

I propose sending you a paper on some of my histological work as it contains some hints for working that may prove useful to your son. It will be printed in a day or two.

The hint you gave me about the hair is very valuable. Have the whiskers of the felidae ever been fully worked out? If not I shall include them.

Yours faithfully

Lawson Tait.

Obviously Tait had not known that Darwin had already reported a pepsine-like substance in the secretion of Drosera but believed he was himself on the track of something quite original. Darwin was becoming a trifle overwhelmed with all this information and he wrote on June 13th indicating that he had already completed the chapters on Drosera in his new book and that he could not use any new observations by Tait. However, he wrote to Tait two days later in an encouraging way: "Your separation of the ferments, seems a capital discovery."

Tait replied on June 16th and sent Darwin a paper on insectivorous plants which he had given in Birmingham. Next day there was another letter describing his complete absorption in his botanical research, "I am so full of my insectivorous plants that I cannot help writing about them, their interest is so intense!" Tait was waiting impatiently for Darwin's book on insectivorous plants to come out and he was able to read it early in July. (c)

July 15 (1875)

My Dear Sir,

I have finished the book and gone over some of the ground new to me. The evidence of absorption is overwhelming and your discovery of "aggregation" alone is enough to immortalise you. I have to review the book for the Spectator so that there you will see my opinions more at length. I have also announced "Insectivorous Plants" as the subject of my Aug. annual lecture at the Sunday Society, St. George's Hall, Langham Place.

There are one or two points where I do not think you are yet complete, but I will not weary you with them now.

I am working at Droseria, but am sadly hampered for want of material. We cannot get the D. Binata anywhere.

I shall find the same thing no doubt in the secretion of the Nepenthus to which I have abundant access.

Let me congratulate you on having made as substantial a contribution to biology as any you have yet achieved and a confirmation of "Darwinism" of the most important character.

Yours faithfully

Lawson Tait.

Insectivorous Plants is a detailed study of these peculiar species. The first twelve chapters are devoted to "Drosera Rotundifolia or the Common Sundew." Darwin had conducted countless experiments to determine the function of the tentacles of the flytrap and had demonstrated their sensitivity to the lightest touch, to foodstuffs, insects, seeds and chemicals. The effects even of chloroform and ether had been studied. He had analysed the ferments produced by the plant and appreciated the fact that stimulation of the tentacles resulted in an acid secretion in which a pepsin-like ferment could digest nitrogenous materials. He had a lot of help in these experiments from his great friend the botanist Hooker, from Dr. Burdon Sanderson and from various chemists with whom he was acquainted. The remaining chapters of the book deal in less detail with other insectivorous plants such as the common Butterwort (Pinguecula) and the rarer Venus Flytrap (Dioneae). Darwin acknowledged Tait's congratulary letter promptly. (c)

17 July (1875)

My Dear Sir,

I thank you for your extremely kind note—I did not answer, as you told me I might not, your former notes to Abinger, as I was quite worn out—I wish I could help you about D. Binate, but I hardly know Lady D. Nevill well enough to borrow plants for a third party —You are aware that Dr. Hooker has worked hard at Nepenthes and will soon publish......

In Haste

Yours sincerely

Ch. Darwin

Darwin had been given botanical specimens by Lady Dorothy Nevill but he did not feel he could arrange this for Tait. The latter was now working hard at the analysis of ferments in fly-catchers such as the pitcher plant (Nepenthe) and announced some success in his next letter. (a)

July 19 (1875)

My Dear Sir,

I have succeeded in separating the ferment of the Nepenthe secretion.

I think the enclosed note may interest you: and if you think it worth publishing will you kindly forward it to *Nature* as Mr. Lockyer has asked me for something on the subject.

Please don't trouble to acknowledge it if it is satisfactory.

Yours faithfully

Lawson Tait.

The note was entitled "Insectivorous Plants" and Darwin sent it on to *Nature.* (c)

July 20 (1875)

My Dear Sir,

I despatched of course your article—I read it rather hurriedly to catch morning post. I will read it deliberately when published. If you have succeeded in separating the ferment the fact is manifestly most important. Did you try whether the fluid from pitchers with no animal matter could digest? This I think ought to have been done to prove that there was ferment in its fluid.....

Yours sincerely

Ch. Darwin

Tait reported in his article experiments on Drosera by which he had confirmed Darwin's observation that the leaves of this plant had considerable absorptive properties. He also described his success in separating a pepsine-like substance and how he had tested its digestive powers.

On July 21 Tait sent Darwin some specimens of abnormal growth of his plants, which he considered as examples of parthenogenesis. Next day a somewhat formal acknowledgement came in the hand of Francis Darwin, one of Charles Darwin's sons. There was just a hint that the expert now felt that Tait's experiments were getting a little out of hand! But Darwin apparently wrote in a more encouraging vein some time in the next few weeks. The irrepressible Tait replied: (a)

Aug. 16 1875

My Dear Sir,

I cannot tell you how much your kind letter has gratified me.

That the *unopened* pitchers of the Nepenthes do contain the ferment *sometimes* is indisputable: and after all not more wonderful than that the gastric mucous membrane always contains pepsine, the amount being increased by the presence of food.

The whole question wants very carefully going over and it is my intention to give some time to it as soon as a run of ovariotomies is over with which I have been engaged. These cases are such a terrible strain that I am always unable to do anything else when I have a number. Then I see my way to quite a book on tails which will be sure to interest the public, as I find my little paper on the cat has made quite a sensation.

I trust you will take really a long rest. How you can do such work as you get through is to me a marvel. I stayed a day with Dr. Andrew Clark at his country place a short time ago and was delighted to hear him speak encouragingly of your health.

Yours sincerely
Lawson Tait.

The paper on the cat was probably the one already mentioned (p. 111).[10] He did not get round to writing a book on tails. His mind was never still and in his next letter he is on to yet another subject! (a)

Sep. 7. (1875)

My Dear Sir,

I am engaged in working out a curious speculation as to the origin of the peculiarities of our moral nature, tracing them from the common origin of parental assistance to the young in the struggle for existence. I propose making it the subject of my introductory lecture to my biology class next month.

Do you know of any earlier instances of parental protection than that of the stickleback?

Spiders don't?
Nor ants?
Anything about vertebrates?

Yours ever

Lawson Tait.

Darwin obliged at once with a quick answer confirming that the maternal instinct was strong in earwigs, starfishes, spiders, sticklebacks and some other fish. But this was a side issue and now Tait was anxious to produce a more elaborate report of his experiments on the insectivorous plants. He asked for Darwin's help in publishing the paper. Meanwhile the paper on the umbilical cord, although presented to the Royal Society, had not brought the hoped for reward or a Fellowship.(a)

Oct. 11 1875

My Dear Sir,

I have a short paper in hand on "The glandular structure and its function in pitcher plants".

Would you favour me by presenting it to the Royal Society for me? I would ask Dr. Hooker, but I do not know him. I am going over the question of the digestion principle but am far from being settled about it. Its presence is essential, but the presence of the acid is far more important.

Yours faithfully

Lawson Tait.

By November Tait thought he had made a considerable breakthrough in his experiments and he communicated his results to Darwin. (a)

Nov. 6th (1875)

My Dear Sir,

I have made a very curious discovery within the last few days. My "Droserin" is a compound substance containing the digestive principle which I propose to designate by that name and another substance which kills the flies by enabling the water to enter their tracheae.

Plain water does not wet flies. They swim for days on its surface. But water containing this substance wets and kills flies in a few minutes.

What shall I call it? I wish your name would allow its being "coined" into "Darwinin".

I have furbished up my Greek to get a term descriptive of its peculiar properties, but I am at a loss.

This substance also accounts for the never drying nature of the secretion.

Yours ever

Lawson Tait.

We do not know Darwin's reaction to the suggestion that the ferment should be named after him, but he continued to acknowledge Tait's letters and to supply numerous references. An elaborate paper was now in preparation for presentation to the Royal Society, and Tait reveals high hopes of its success. (a)

Nov. 20 (1875)

My Dear Sir,

I have just finished my paper.
It remains to be fair copied, but that will take only a few days. It is longer than I expected, facts have such a habit of accumulating, but I have made it as succinct as possible.

Shall I send it to you or to the Society? In the event of your wanting to read it might I suggest that I could save you the labour by reading it to you. I shall be in town on Friday night having to lecture on Sunday, and I could bring it with me to Down on Saturday forenoon and read it to you. I need not say how much I should like to know your opinion of it. I think I could read it in an hour to you but I trust you will not bore yourself with it. The abstract which will accompany it will give you most of the conclusions.

Yours truly

Lawson Tait.

There was no invitation to Down but in due course Darwin did read the paper and sent it to the Royal Society. There are two puzzling aspects of all this. Firstly, Darwin must have realised that Tait's work was rather scrappy and that many of the findings had already been published by Darwin himself (in *Insectivorous Plants*). Secondly, Tait *had* read Darwin's monograph and he should have realised that in this field he could scarcely be seen as a serious competitor. We may only conjecture that Darwin did not read the paper very carefully. If he *was* aware of its deficiencies then perhaps it was a little ill-judged that he should have passed it to the Royal Society. There is a hint that he was doubtful about the validity of Tait's chemical evidence. There is confirmation too that on account of one of his bouts of ill health he did not study the paper in detail. (a)

Nov. 27th (1875)

My Dear Sir,

I have looked through the whole of your paper but have not read it very carefully as I have been unwell and confined to bed and now a pile of proofs is waiting for correction. Your paper seems to me, as far as I can judge a very important contribution to science, and I hope that your chemical observations which must have been extremely difficult will be hereafter confirmed. It seems a great anomaly the two substances with an acid should be requisite for digestion. I will despatch your paper registered tomorrow to the R. Soc.

My Dear Sir
Yours faithfully
Ch. Darwin.

Tait wrote on Nov. 29th thanking Darwin for his help and admitting that the chemical part of the paper was weak because of his lack of experience. Now he had to wait for the verdict. He knew that his election as a Fellow of the Royal Society must depend largely on the reception of his work. His experiments on the insectivorous plants were now abandoned and he turned to other subjects such as his views on survival of the fittest insofar as civilised humans were concerned. He wrote at length on this subject to Darwin on Feb. 21 1876. A week later there was a letter of great interest to Darwin. Tait at this time believed that if a supernumerary digit was amputated in an infant the digit might grow again. Paget had given Darwin evidence to the contrary. Darwin wrote on March 10 about this matter. (c)

March 20 1876

My Dear Sir,

Sir J. Paget has not published on the subject, but took extraordinary trouble in corresponding with various eminent surgeons and writing to me. He gave me particulars of some degree of regrowth especially of the humerus but disbelieves in a digit ever being reproduced.

He goes on so far as to suspect that when even a nail is reproduced part of the matrix has been left; but I cannot avoid thinking that he is in this respect over sceptical. I sent him full particulars and tracings of the two cases which had been communicated to me.

I send by this post Dr. Rudinger's essay which I advise you to read.

I think your intention of amputating the extra digit of a kitten is an excellent idea. Could not you try also on a Dorking fowl. I suppose you could keep the amputated little toe in spirits; and then if there were regrowths you could give drawings of the bones of the first digit and of the regrowth. I would suggest your amputating one of the ordinary toes at the same time as a control experiment.

I am glad you are examining tail-less animals, but it would not be worth-while to send me the specimens, as I have not sufficient knowledge and am much engaged with other subjects.

I fear that you will fail about regrowth, but if you can prove it the discovery will be an interesting one.

My dear Sir

Yours sincerely

Ch. Darwin.

The discussion continued and Tait became a little obstinate in his opinions. He wrote on March 27th "It seems to me that the reproduction of lost parts in an early stage follows as a matter of course, if the process of evolution really takes place. . . . I am quite certain of it and mean to work it out."

Some time in early April the verdict on Tait's paper on insectivorous plants came through. It was completely unfavourable and it was a great disappointment. Tait's immediate impulse was to write to Darwin; it was a rather abject and somewhat pathetic letter. (a)

April 25 (1876)

My Dear Sir,

I do not know in which terms to make my apology for having placed you in so objectionable a position, as to be sponsor for a rejected paper.

The lesson to me is a severe one, but one to be profited by and for the future I shall not venture in to subjects where even my elementary knowledge seems deficient. The snubbing about the use of the terms seems from the pencilled remarks of the referee to be thoroughly deserved, and if you know who he is, I should be obliged if you would let him know this. . . .

Yours truly

Lawson Tait.

Darwin eventually sent Tait an extract of the referee's report and there was severe criticism of the techniques used and of the interpretation of the chemical analysis. It was all too clear that Tait had not informed himself completely of the literature on his subject and that he lacked the expertise to carry out the chemical methods involved. Perhaps with so much more pressing work on his hands he had been careless, in too much of a hurry and too ready to fit his results into his preconceived theories. He did not attempt much further experimental work of this type.[11] After this somewhat unfortunate episode letters continued to be exchanged on a variety of subjects. Tait remained a fervent disciple of Darwin and was determined that the world should recognise that he was the greatest scientist of the age. In 1876 Tait was President of the Birmingham Natural History Society. He wrote to Darwin on August 4th, asking permission to add his name to the roll of Honorary Members. He took the opportunity of sending some recent papers he had written. Darwin accepted the honour graciously and commented on the papers. (c)

Aug. 6. 76

My Dear Sir,

I shall feel much pleasure and honour if I am elected one of your members and I beg you to return on your part my best thanks to your Society.

I read with interest the articles which you were so good as to send me and I agree with the greater part–Under a theological point of view, I cannot quite agree that the origin of evil is explained by Survival.

Why should a thumb cut cause tetanus, or childbirth—or parasitic works cause so much suffering? Why was not man formed with sympathies extending beyond his own tribe, so that murder would have been a crime from the earliest period?

I am glad that you have not given up polydactylism. -

Very dear Sir

Yours faithfully

Ch. Darwin.

Darwin refers in his letter to "The Evolution of Our Moral Life," a paper contributed by Tait to the *Birmingham Examiner.* In this essay Tait attempted to show how "the mental and moral state of man, his civilisation and culture in the arts and sciences, his religions and aspirations for a higher state" might be understood from evolutionary theory. He drew a parallel between the vestigial organs found in man or in animals and the survival of old customs and traditions in religious and social life, describing such survivals as "the fossils of Anthropology." He discussed the theory of primitive good and the growth of evil. A sin such as murder he explained by reversion of type to primitive man or even to an animal state. The social instincts he saw as simple evolutionary developments from animal instincts. His final message was that biological studies were neither atheistic nor irreligious but, on the contrary, could lead to humility and true religion; the understand of good and evil was to come from the "grand simplicity and universal influence of the Law of Evolution."

Having had some comment from Darwin on these philosophical and religious questions Tait wrote two days later to expand on his notions of the origin of diseases; once more he insisted that such questions could be solved by applying Darwin's evolutionary principles. (a)

Aug. 8 '76.

My Dear Sir

Thanks for your prompt and kind compliance with my wish.

I trust you will forgive me saying that your objection seems to me to arise from mixing up the idea of moral evil with physical evil or suffering. Strange though it may seem the second question seems to me the simpler of the two.

I will not at present take up your time with my notions on the origin of diseases, but I am gradually framing a theory by which it will be brought under the great rule of evolution. But the question is so complicated that it merits the most cautious handling and the better plan would be to follow the example of Fritz Müller and take one disease and work out the proof of your theory there as he did in the Crustaceans.

But unfortunately we do not know the natural history of any one disease! An awful [indecipherable], hindering the progress of Medical Science in every direction.

I purpose to take syphilis as my example because we know more about it than about any other disease.....

But then it is a subject we cannot make acceptable to the public. Yet the sexual question is the most important field for our studies and the process of evolution.

Yours faithfully

Lawson Tait.

For some time Tait continued in his attempt to simplify the classification and understanding of diseases and to explain their origin by an application of evolutionary theory. No more is heard of his proposed intensive study of syphilis and indeed this was a rather complicated, ill-defined disease to choose for any such research. Next year he wrote again to Darwin seeking criticism of his latest book. (a)

Jan 16 1877

My Dear Sir,

If our views on Evolution are sound it seems to me that they must include many explanations of the diseased processes of man. I am writing a book on diseases of women and am trying to borrow light from the *Descent of Man.* I send two or three proof sheets containing a sample and though I know how you hesitate to express an opinion on a matter out of the lines of your experiences, if you can see your way to criticise (in general terms(my views, I should like to know your opinion.

I have another matter in which I think I have done better than in the present case, hermaphroditism, which I would like to submit to you in a few days.

"Cross Fertilisation" is splendid. I have just published a review for the *Spectator.*

Yours truly

Lawson Tait

Darwin answered briefly and agreed with all that Tait had written. The discussion went on during February in further letters and in due course Tait sent a copy of his *Diseases of Women.* Darwin read some of the book with interest and was pleased at some brief references to his own work. (c)

June 15 (1887)

My Dear Sir,

Your note and kind present of your work on the Diseases of Women has been forwarded to me here where I am staying for a little change and rest—I have read the interesting passages to which you refer me, and will hereafter look at some other portions of your book. You never fail to honour me much more than I deserve.

My dear Sir

Yours very faithfully

Charles Darwin

P.S. I was much interested by your letter on a cat rearing chickens, which is the converse case of a hen rearing young ferrets, as described by Romanes some time ago in Nature. What a wonderful instinct is the maternal one!

In December 1877 Tait wrote to Darwin on a new subject, the sacrococcygeal dimple; it was rather a scribbled and untidy letter with some crude drawings. (a)

Dec. 31 1877

My Dear Sir

I believe I have made a discovery which will greatly interest you. It is no less than the method by which tails are lost and I have found evidence of the process in man which I think will prove as weighty as "Darwin's ear" is in another direction.

It is too long a matter for me to go into now but let me merely say that the process is the occurrence of spina bifida and the remnant in man of the process consists of depression of the skin over the point of the coccyx and its union (by fascial adhesion) to the posterior surface of the tip bone. I have been engaged all morning in making casts of the depressions in a family of children who have it marked in all and very marked in one. The mother has it. The very marked one I try to give you an idea in the diagram. The depression is tubular and quite half an inch deep.

Yours truly

Lawson Tait.

[P.S.] I think it quite on a par with the pharyngeal fistula which indicates the lost branchial opening and the labial furrow which shows the lost hare lip.

L.T.

The condition which Tait described in this letter is a common one but he was jumping to a rather ill-considered conclusion when he suggested that this dimple in the region of the coccyx was indicative of a lost tail. Tait read a paper at the British Association meeting in Dublin in August 1878 entitled: "Note on the Occurrence of a Sacral Dimple and its Possible Significance". He argued that tailed vertebrates might produce offspring with the deficiency of the lower spinal column known as spina bifida and that this deficiency might destroy the foetal tail at an early stage of growth, with a resultant dimple or scar in the sacral region. His argument was not put forward very convincingly and his audience, the Section of Anatomy, did not accept it very readily.

The proceedings of the association were fully reported by the Dublin press and Tait's paper was commented on adversely because it was considered quite disgraceful to submit hundreds of patients (as Tait described) in a women's hospital to search for this anomaly out of mere curiosity! There was even a doggerel verse, "Lines on a Sacral Dimple", printed and distributed in Birmingham. Tait was described in uncomplimentary terms:[12]

A few Surgeons in this town
Thought it would be pleasant
To have a hospital for women
Which was opened in the Crescent.

. . . . .

A Gorilla was appointed
With long hair down his back
His name I will not mention
It might put you on his track.

. . . . .

And when these women go
Examined by him to be,
He makes statistics of the place
Where he says tails ought to be.

. . . . .

These poor women wonder now,
And indeed feel quite indignant,
Why he should so desire to see
Their sacro-coccygeal ligament.

. . . . .

Unless indeed a wife has he
And a long tail she has got
His great propensity is to know
If all women have tails, or not.

. . . . .

After 1878 Tait's correspondence with Darwin almost ceased as far as the exchange of scientific information was concerned. He gave a lecture to the Birmingham Philosophical Society in 1878 on the "Evolution of the Sense of Hearing" and this was amongst the last of his studies on evolution. He was still active in his support of Darwin and he wrote to him at the beginning of 1880. (a)

Jan. 12 1880

My Dear Sir,

This day month is your birthday and we propose here to have a "Darwin Festival" on a small scale probably, but as hearty and as large as we can secure. May I ask if you would be willing to accept some little expression of our gratitude for your work – say an illuminated address or something of the kind? Also can you refer me to any biographical notices beyond that of "Men of the Time" and Dublin University Magazine? The date in question is the completion of your 70th year is it not? – or rather the day before is – and that your 71st birthday.

Our Philosophical Society meets that day, therefore arises the opportunity.

Yours truly
Lawson Tait.

Darwin was by this time a rather tired old man. He replied the next day. "The honour which you propose is a great one," he wrote. "But would it not be better to wait until I am in my grave?" However, he was made an Honorary Member of the Philosophical Society. Tait wrote on January 18th to confirm this. He had composed the address and sent a rough copy for approval with the comment: (a)

> . . . . We desire to do this, not only for the honouring of a man whom we regard as the head of the scientific world but to give a fillip to the removal of that singular terror which the word "Darwin" excites in the minds of religionists and other uneducated people that is the bulk of the community . . . .

Darwin was pleased with the address: "according to my judgement no one could possibly have written it in better taste." Later in the year on July 15th Tait wrote of the intention of the Birmingham Naturalists' Society to establish a "Charles Darwin Prize" for local observation or research of an original character. He asked for a contribution towards a research fund. Darwin responded generously with £25. In due course a medal was struck with an excellent likeness of Darwin executed by Joseph Moore. There is some uncertainty as to whether or not the medal was ever awarded.

In 1881 Tait did communicate once more on a scientific matter. (c)

July 29 1881

My Dear Sir,

I have just read your paper on "Inheritance".

Will you forgive me if I point out two possibilities of fallacy in it? I am sure you will.

The case of the nails is in all probability a case of syphilis, as the peculiarity died out in the [?] generation with succeeding children. The disease is well known to be a variety of tertiary syphilis and if such a case had appeared in a medical journal I think it would have unquestionably have been set down as due to that cause.

Guinea pigs: Brown-Sequard's observations are quite worthless, for under certain circumstances of diet every other guinea pig has epilepsy. I have kept them for years by the hundred and I could have epilepsy abundant or not as I liked by giving them moist or dry food and varieties.

It was not hereditary and it—as often as not—could be induced on irritation of the "epileptic regions of B.S." It certainly had nothing to do with division of the cord or of the sciatic nerves.

I have published all this somewhere but I cannot recall it.

Yours faithfully

Lawson Tait.

The tone is just a little peremptory. In earlier years Tait wrote to Darwin as would a humble student to his master. This letter is rather reminiscent of those with which Tait was accustomed to castigate his medical colleagues. Perhaps it is significant that no reply survives and indeed none may have been sent.

The last known letter from Darwin to Tait was early in 1882. It was short and rather sad. (c)

Feb. 13 1882

My Dear Sir,

I must write one line to thank you and Mrs. Tait for your very kind note on my birthday.

I feel I am a very old man and my course is nearly run.

I remain,

Yours very sincerely

Ch. Darwin.

On March 30, 1882 Francis Darwin acknowledged the receipt of a medal (probably a copy of the Prize medal prepared in 1880). He thanked Tait for his kind expressions about his father's health. There had been a steady decline in the previous three years and Darwin had lost his zest for scientific investigation. Late in February there were recurrent cardiac attacks and on April 19, 1882, he died.

Lawson Tait's last significant public reference to Darwin and his work was in his Presidential Address to the Birmingham Philosophical Society in October 1885. He reminded his audience of his early support of Darwin and the contribution he himself had made in his paper to the *Dublin Journal* in 1869. He recalled how this paper had involved him in much adverse criticism. He said, "There is not much danger now in almost any part of England in a man being a follower of the Darwinian philosophy, but fifteen years ago it was dangerous in most places, and not very popular even here." With perhaps some exaggeration Tait stated, "I have lived to see a few of the broad principles which I attempted to lay down accepted as part of the creed of the modern evolutionists. In fact I have lived to see them stolen and brought out as new and original views by men who were virulent opponents of Darwin at the time I wrote them. . . ." Tait was unfortunately now tending to write papers and give addresses in which he had nothing very new to offer, serving up old material and often querulously suggesting that his ideas had either been neglected or plagiarised. The address consisted very largely of lengthy quotations from the Dublin paper of 1869 and from his article in the *Birmingham Examiner* of 1876. He had really nothing new to say.

We must assess fairly Tait's involvement in one of the greatest scientific controversies of the age. He had the curiosity and intelligence to study Darwin's works when they first appeared, despite the fact that he breathed an atmosphere in which support to Darwin bordered on heresy. He at once appreciated the significance of the new theory of evolution. As a young surgeon he risked rejection in academic and other circles because of his advanced views. As an established surgeon with little spare time he was prepared to devote much energy to experimental work which was difficult and tedious but from which he genuinely hoped to add something in support of Darwin's theories. He found time also to read widely on scientific subjects outside medicine, believing that disease processes might be better understood—and managed—by application of the new biology.

As things turned out, his experimental research was rather a failure. From his rather sad letter to Darwin, when he heard that his work on insectivorous plants had not been accepted by the Royal Society, he said he was aware that he was not really equipped to carry out the experiments he described. It was something to have tried, but a subsequent verdict that "he was no scientist" is probably correct. Unsuccessful though this particular venture might have been, we cannot but admire his enthusiasm, and it would be unkind to suggest that he undertook this research only to have a better chance of being awarded an F.R.S.

In 1875 Darwin had reached a stage in his career which allowed him to sit back philosophically and accept the idea that his own great contribution was not entirely original but owed much to others. So he was generous to a young enthusiast like Tait and gave him what seems in retrospect to have been almost excessive encouragement. Before Darwin had published the *Origin* his ideas had been gestating for twenty-five years; he must have recognised in Tait an amateur scientist given to hasty and at times obstinate conclusions, and yet he gave him his support.

In retrospect, Tait always spoke of his friendship with Darwin as one of the most important things in his life and he saw in him a constant source of inspiration. Darwin was his hero.

CHAPTER VIII

The Years of Success and Influence

In 1878 the Women's Hospital was transferred to a new building at Sparkhill and four years later Lawson Tait moved from his house in Great Charles Street. He purchased numbers seven, eight and nine of the Crescent, the original site of the Women's Hospital. He lived in number seven, the other two houses being remodelled for use as a private hospital.[1] While most of his operative work in the next years was done either in the new Women's Hospital or at the Crescent, he travelled all over the British Isles to see patients; when necessary, he operated in their homes, although he preferred to work in a hospital.

The organisation of Tait's private hospital interested his numerous visitors greatly and many Americans recorded their impressions. Professor Robinson of Chicago gave the following account in 1892:[2]

> Mr. Tait sustains a private hospital for the treatment of his surgical patients. This hospital bears evidence of good ventilation and plumbing. . . . The furniture of the hospital is simple and not excessive. . . . He keeps twenty-five beds which are generally full. . . . He keeps twelve nurses in his private hospital. He selects young and intelligent women for nurses and then he trains them in his private hospital. He seems desirous that they shall be neat, cheerful and interested in their work. It is a matter of surprise what eagerness one of these nurses will manifest in trying to get a case well who has been put in her charge. Each nurse counts, sadly, her death records and she will often announce with pride how many months she has nursed patients without a single death. . . . A nurse is given charge of a patient on whom abdominal section has been performed and she sits up with her without sleep in severe cases, and the nurse is not allowed to leave her for five days. After that the patient is left for short intervals but a bell string is close to the patient's hand . . . connected with an electrical apparatus in the dining room. The operation is done in the patient's room where she will remain. Mr. Tait does not have a single operating room. A board about eighteen inches wide is laid on two 'horses' for a table. As soon as his assistant puts the patient to sleep one of the nurses calls Mr. Tait. . . . He enters the room and at a glance generally satisfies himself if all things are in readiness. . . .

> Mr. Tait employs a lady superintendent in his hospital who supervises in general and relieves him from its care. His hospital is the outcome of many years of discipline. . . . He has the capacity to make paid labour serviceable. . . . Paid labour relieves him from the preparation of patient or instruments. It takes away the anxious care of after treatment. He keeps a secretary who does his correspondence with a typewriter. When Mr. Tait wishes to write an article or a letter he simply talks it off to his secretary and she takes it down in shorthand.

Professor Robinson was obviously impressed by this efficent organisation and his observations reveal how much of Tait's surgical success was due to the high quality of nursing care given to his patients and to the strict isolation which avoided cross-infection, whether in the ward or the theatre. Vander Veer, Professor of Surgery in New York, was another American much impressed by Tait's private hospital:[3]

> His hospital is a model of all that one could wish regarding quietness, cleanliness and perfect system, not only in nursing but in everything. . . .
>
> He selects young, intelligent and prepossessing women whom he trains for the work he so much enjoys and they in their desire to please become true enthusiasts in the struggle to save life. He will not have morose, untidy or homely women for nurses. . . .
>
> Rooms are thoroughly cleansed after each patient leaves and no display is made of any particular antiseptic in so doing. Nurses and attendants go about with cheerful faces but no noise. Mr. Tait himself when going through the rooms visiting makes but few remarks aside from that which is required in dictating treatment, etc., and although a man who enjoys a well-told story and general conversation, indulges in no talk here . . . . his own dwelling adjoins his hospital and communicates with it and when a case goes badly he is promptly on hand trusting to no one else to right matters. In his operations he has a lady physician to administer the anaesthetic . . . and one male assistant whose position is directly opposite him and yet who is seldom allowed to handle any of the sponges or instruments, only assisting when the abdominal walls are being opened and in ligating the pedicle, appendages or adhesions. . . .

Working in this highly efficient environment at the peak of his career what manner of man was Tait? There are many descriptions of him; perhaps those of the American visitors are particularly relevant, since they were usually meeting Tait for the first time and carried away with them very distinct and unbiassed impressions. Professor Robinson writes:

> Personally Tait is a short, stout man. . . . He has a large head covered with dark iron-gray hair. He wears only small side whiskers. He speaks moderately quick, and thinks very rapidly. In operating when complications arise he makes quick decisions and then quickly executes them without hesitation. He is very reticent and quiet while at work, but when not engaged, is often talkative and enjoys a well told story. He has a large fund of humorous and witty stories which he can relate in the most pointed style. He is a good entertainer at dinners. . . . He is an inveterate reader and reads in his carriage and in trains. He is fond of good theatres and frequently attends them. . . .
>
> He spends much of his time travelling to operate in Great Britain and other countries. He was a great admirer of the celebrated surgeon Syme and uses little short bladed knives and drives heavy gray horses just as that operator did. Mr. Tait's heavy gray span with their vigorous action are well known in Birmingham.

Of Tait's successive assistants two in particular give detailed pictures of their master. William Stewart McKay (1866-1948), his first biographer, came from Australia in 1891 and was with Tait for a year. McKay returned to Sydney to practise as a gynaecologist. He became an able surgeon but never attained to a consultant post in one of the more important teaching hospitals. When he died it was recorded in his obituary that his short association with Tait had had a lifelong influence, but "an influence for good and some evil."[4] McKay had Tait's aggressiveness, squandering his fortune recklessly on the race-course. Like Tait, he stood out as a person of great originality and scholarship in many subjects outside the field of medicine.

McKay came to England well aware of Tait's reputation, and determined to study under him. On his arrival in London he met a young American who had tried to get an interview with Tait but had failed (Tait had become a little tired of the many Americans who wanted to work with him). Undeterred, McKay telegraphed Tait to say that he was coming to see him. When he arrived in Birmingham he was admitted to his study:[5]

> . . .the door opened, a short man with a huge head, long hair, side whiskers and dressed in a velvet coat entered the room. I glanced at him but the individual was so unlike what I imagined Lawson Tait

> would actually be that I said nothing. However he did not leave me long in doubt for he said in a voice that was anything but pleasant, "Well do you want to see me?" I was so flabbergasted but managed to say "I would like to see Dr. Lawson Tait". "There is no *Dr.* Lawson Tait here! If you want to see *Mr.* Lawson Tait follow me".
>
> I followed him into his consulting room and sat down in an easy chair – he did not seat himself, he stood by his desk, and said, "Well, what do you want?" I looked up at Tait and said "I have come from Australia to learn Gynaecology and they tell me you know most about it and I thought I'd come and ask you to take me on as your assistant", and I looked and smiled at him. (He later told me he was greatly taken by my beautiful teeth) . . . . I watched his face for it exhibited a look of utter surprise. Then he burst out laughing and he laughed and laughed: he seemed to think it was a splendid joke, so I thought I better join in and we both laughed. Then he said, "That is the best thing I've heard for many a day" . . . .he put his hand on my shoulder and said "I'll take you as my assistant, just for the fun of the thing."

It was all very typical of Tait's unpredictable character and of his quick decisions. He appreciated the Australian's frankness and determination. McKay remained with Tait, absorbing all his teaching, becoming one of his most faithful disciples, and looking back on this day in August 1891 as the most eventful of his life. There was much hard work, but there were relaxations and they became close friends. The young assistant accompanied the Taits on frequent excursions to their country house in the New Forest or to their houseboat on the river Avon at Cropthorne. On such trips business was combined with pleasure, all of it being done in style:

> When I had been a short time with Tait he received a telegram asking him to go and perform an urgent operation . . . . the bags of instruments were soon ready and we left by the first train: Dr. Ambler, a friend of Tait, going with us to give the anaesthetic. Tait had ordered a first class carriage to be reserved for us as we had to go to Bournemouth. After we started he produced a basket with cold grouse and wine and we lunched and smoked until the long journey was over at six o'clock. We proceeded to the patient's home where the medical attendant awaited us and Tait decided it was a case of ruptured tubal pregnancy and said he would operate at once.

The operation was completed successfully although a fine carpet on the bedroom floor was ruined by the blood which dripped from the makeshift table. McKay was worried about this and thought Tait rather careless. The latter reassured him: "The husband of the patient is the largest manufacturer of carpets in England and he won't bother as long as his wife is saved." Afterwards they all relaxed at Buskett Fletchwood in the New Forest. It was the first of many such excursions:

> Let me first explain that Tait was married and was very fond of his very pretty wife but his one sorrow was this, that they had no children. Perhaps it was this fact that made him act so kindly towards me.
>
> . . . . he was not always in an amiable mood at his house in Birmingham: while he was always "jolly as a sandboy" once he was in the country.
>
> If we were driving along we passed an old building or an old church he would pull up and Mrs. Tait would hold the reins while we went to the building and Tait gave me a lecture on the particular variety of architecture at which we were looking. . . .
>
> Then he adopted another plan which was equally as pleasant, for if he was invited to operate in some part of England he would arrange that the operation should be done on the Saturday morning and we would proceed to the destination on Friday afternoon by train. On these trips Tait was at his best, for being very fond of large fees, after he had pocketed the fee on Saturday he would be in the best of tempers. . . .
>
> I well remember the first of these trips, to the West Riding of Yorkshire: the operation was completed, the local practitioner took charge, while we departed in a carriage and had a long and delightful drive for two days by Bolton Castle, where I was told Mary Stuart had been imprisoned, through Wensleydale past Gervaux Abbey, on to York. What a treat in the countryside of England, with its exquisite trees, to an Australian.
>
> What I used to like was to get Tait to speak about the famous men he had known. Sitting round a peat fire in his home in the New Forest – how he loved a good dinner – and mellowed by some of his superb wines which he had been collecting for years, he was always ready to tell you anything he could. On the 24th of August, it being my birthday, he gave us a splendid dinner and opened a bottle of champagne that the Czar of Russia had given him. It was a beautiful wine, Gratz, but too sweet. Tait had operated on the Czar's old physician for gall-stones, the Czar had paid him £1,000 for the operation.
>
> Next to these weekend trips the Wednesday night suppers which Tait gave to leading actors . . . . Tait had a penchant for well-known

actors and actresses and every Wednesday evening he made a point of having some of the principals to supper; among those that came were Henry Irving and Ellen Terry, Beerbohm Tree, Wilson Barret and others. . . . I well remember Wilson Barret telling a story at supper. He said that once in Edinburgh he was playing Hamlet and the actor that played "The Ghost" fell ill at the last minute. He had no understudy and he was in a fix. Then one of the theatre hands said he had a friend that had played the ghost. Barret found him word perfect – the play began and all went well until the Ghost appearing he was recognised immediately by some friends in the gallery as he was a *butcher* and they sang out "Hie Jock what price steak today?" The play could not go on as Jock came forward and shaking his fist at his friends said "If yee don't shut up I'll up and trample the tripes out of yee!", and after this all went well!

While in the biographies of the notable actors and actresses who dined with Tait in Birmingham when they played in that city his name scarcely appears, it does seem that Tait did get to know Sir Henry Irving well. In 1892 Lawrence, Sir Henry's second son, while in Dublin, attempted suicide by shooting himself through the chest. Tait was summoned at once from Birmingham. He found that Lawrence had survived his injury, complimented the Irish doctors on their treatment and was able to reassure Sir Henry of his son's recovery.[6]

In his biography of Tait, McKay recalls many other incidents which illuminate Tait's way of life and his character in general. He impressed on his pupil the way in which men like Lister, Syme, Fergusson and Simpson, operating without the benefit of anaesthesia, acquired a dexterity which in Tait's opinion could never be equalled. McKay records: "Syme had been his teacher; Liston he only knew by report: Fergusson he had little or nothing to do with, but Simpson had been his friend, and was, I have little doubt, his father." Tait spoke in admiration of the American Marion Sims. Of some British contemporaries, particularly lister and Spencer Wells, he was invariably critical and vehemently so.

Christopher Martin (1866-1933) was Tait's pupil and then his assistant from 1889 onwards. He was appointed consultant in the Women's Hospital in 1890 and continued in Birmingham as a gynaecologist of some distinction.[7] After qualification in Edinburgh he had come with an introduction to Tait from Professor Alexander Simpson, the nephew of Sir James. Within a week of his arrival in Birmingham Martin fell ill and Tait kindly took him to convalesce at his home in the New Forest.

In 1891 Martin became Tait's partner and Charles, his brother, Tait's secretary. In a short memoir of Tait Martin describes him: [8]

> Once seen he was not easily forgotten. He was a short stout man, with a magnificent head, corpulent body, podgy legs, and small hands and feet. Some one described him as "a man with the body of Bacchus and the head of Jove." He had a small finely shaped mouth, a firm chin, and eyes which had a wonderful power of fascination. His voice was soft and musical – I have heard him sing sweetly: but when enraged he could roar like a lion. He had a very big head – he took 8 in hats – a fine head of hair, just beginning to turn grey.

The picture is not entirely flattering, for the years were beginning to take their toll of Tait. Once more the resemblances to Simpson are apparent and indeed the detail "the head of Jove" had been applied to Simpson. Martin, incidentally, did not believe that Tait was Simpson's natural son. That Tait was a man not easily forgotten by those who knew him is clear from Martin's appraisal:

> He was a man of great force of character and by his personal magnetism dominated those with whom he came in contact – certainly all in his service. They worshipped him and would do anything for him. In this respect, as in many others, he resembled Napoleon. He had many interests – inside and outside his profession – many irons in the fire at once. He never spent an idle moment, and the amount of work he got through was marvellous.

Martin records a typical day in Tait's life. He was called at 7 a.m., completed his letters by 8:30 a.m., and operated at the Women's Hospital or at the Crescent in the morning. In the afternoon he saw patients at his consulting room, working with great rapidity. He wasted few words on his patients, telling them briefly what was the matter with them and what should be done. They could take it or leave it. He was no respecter of persons and never toadied to the rich or great. In the evenings there were meetings of the medical societies or of local organisations, lectures and the like, to all of which he contributed vigorously:

> He was very clean in his person, dressed for comfort rather than appearance. . . . In his own house he usually wore a velvet lounge coat . . . . On one occasion a doctor who was a stickler for appearances, called him out to see a county lady. Tait turned up in a lounge coat and soft hat, and the doctor remarked on his unprofessional garb.

Tait got very angry and he growled "Do you want to consult my hat or my brains?" On the other hand, he always insisted that I should be dressed *de rigueur* in frock coat and silk hat. One day I had the temerity to ask him why I could not also wear a soft hat in public like himself and he replied "Because *I* am Lawson Tait, and *you* are only Christopher Martin."

. . . . He was a curious mixture of generosity and Scotch parsimony. While on the one hand he spent lavishly on his pleasures or in the pursuit of his hobbies, he was scrupulously careful over trifles.

. . . He was an able and convincing speaker, ready in retort, quick to see the weak points in his opponents' arguments and clever in conceding his own. . . . He was an ugly enemy: and when he hit he hit hard and did not mind whether it was below or above the belt.

In private life he was a charming companion and it was a pleasure to listen to his conversation. Some of the most interesting hours I ever spent were at his dinner table where he entertained all sorts of guests – Kropotkin the Russian nihilist, John Stuart Blackie of Edinburgh, Alfred Hayes the poet, Toole the actor, Hugh Fraser the diplomatist, Canon O'Sullivan of Solihull and others. It was a treat to listen to them, with their wit and repartee and many stories.

He had a violent temper and, when he let himself go, was like a raging bull. I remember once he got in a passion with a telephone operator: and, as he could not lay hands on her, tore down the instrument from the wall and jumped on it.

Martin, like McKay, describes the weekend excursions and the long drives to consultations in the country. Tait had the useful capacity of sleeping anywhere at any time, so recharging his immense energy:

One Sunday afternoon we were returning via Lichfield and he took me into the cathedral. The evening service was just beginning. When it came to the Magnificat and Nunc Dimittis he stood up and sang lustily in Latin (he remembered the words from his Catholic boyhood): but during prayers and lessons he promptly fell asleep and snored. I kept nudging him to waken him, till he finally growled, "Let's go out", and very glad I was to do so.

Such accounts give a vivid picture of Tait's remarkable energy, his capacity for hard work and his ability to relax when time allowed. His character emerges as an extraordinary mixture of humanity, intellect, curiosity, impetuosity and aggressiveness. He was quite unpredictable in his reactions to people and events. This strange mixture was accepted by those who came under his spell but less readily understood by others. His aggressiveness and surliness were at their worst in his dealings with some of his colleagues. Spencer Wells, at first friendly with him, then simply ignored his taunts and insults over professional matters. Even Tait's gibe, "it would have been better for posterity if Sir Spencer Wells had continued his services in Her Majesty's Navy and had never touched abdominal surgery", remained unanswered. There were some who spoke their minds about Tait. Bland Sutton records that "Tait was a quarrelsome fellow, rough and rude."[9] Gilbert Barling, a Birmingham surgeon who knew Tait well, wrote of "his genius for friendship and hospitality combined with a capacity for quarrelling with his best friends, which made him at times impossible." Dr. Francis Brett Young, who was well informed of the Birmingham medical scene, brings into the novel *Dr. Bradley Remembers* a thinly disguised character obviously based on Tait, namely one "Simpson Lyle, that great, bloated, insolent, foul-mouthed genius – yet you must grant him that."[10] This is a cruel picture which exaggerates darker shades of Tait's character.

In his lifetime Tait was portrayed in another fictional work, *The Star Sapphire,* by Mabel Wilkins. In this minor novel the main character is Culverton Brand, a surgeon owning a private hospital in "Birchampton." Almost certainly the picture is of Tait, far in advance of his profession and consequently greatly disliked by his colleagues. This antagonism is magnified into a national boycott of his pupils and the fruits of his genius gathered only by Americans. "He is a man of contradictions. I have heard him called a genius and a fool, lavish and parsimonious, delightful and hateful. Great operators are generally odd characters, but he is the oddest of them all."[11]

Oliver Wendell Holmes, in his *One Hundred Days in Europe*, records an encounter with Lawson Tait: "As I sat by the side of this great surgeon a question suggested itself to my mind . . . . which would give the most satisfaction to a thoroughly humane and unselfish being, of cultivated intelligence and lively sensibilities: to have written all the plays of Shakespeare . . . . or to have snatched from the jaws of death more than a hundred fellow creatures. . . .?"[12]

The atmosphere created by Tait is revealed by these personal observations; from these and many other sources, we can build up a remarkably complete picture of his domestic life and his interests outside of medicine. His lucrative private practice allowed him to live in considerable luxury; it would also appear that, although he was parsimonious, particularly in his dealings with his assistants, he was not thrifty, for he does not seem to have invested any of his rapidly acquired fortune either for his old age or for his wife's comfort.

There exists no detailed description of his Birmingham home, but the lavish hospitality given there does suggest that it was comfortable and well furnished. He purchased Buskett Fletchwood in the New Forest, near Lyndhurst, in the early eighties.[13] This was a spacious Victorian house with a large conservatory, with extensive and secluded grounds. There is a glimpse of the lavishness of its furnishing in a snapshot of Tait and his wife by a heavily carved rococo spiral pillar, an ornate fireplace and a cabinet full of *objets d'art*. Here Tait accumulated over some 15 years his extraordinary collection of curiosities, ornaments and pictures. He collected things ranging from Chinese and Japanese curios to Roman Catholic and Russian Orthodox pictures, triptychs and crucifixes. Many of his treasures were gifts from grateful patients and many he acquired on his travels abroad. He went to great lengths to bring these home. In Italy he purchased a Della Robbia relief and to get round the laws against exporting works of art he concealed it in a large cheese and so evaded the Customs officer.

Some suggested that he lacked taste, but most of Tait's visitors, and particularly those from America, were impressed by his bizarre collection. One American visitor (Professor Robinson) recalls a visit to Buskett Fletchwood:[14]

> . . . . Mr. Tait remarked to me that when I got into his country seat I would be living in the sixteenth century. The ceiling covering the reception room is made from the timber taken from the room in which Catherine of Aragon was married to Arthur Prince of Wales. Quaint old bureaus, carved chests and ancient looking chairs are found in all the rooms. Pictures and casts, and busts, and horns and old relics of every description may be seen through the house. Hosts of old dishes, porcelaine, rare china ware and many remnants of firearms can be seen. Relics from the chivalry and the tournament are not few. It is a model house, richly furnished. He keeps quite a number of servants to cultivate and improve the estate, which is adorned with fountains, conservatories, hot houses, orchards, lawns, well ordered gardens and walks.

While Tait was intensely curious about all human activities, and remarkably well-informed on the most diverse subjects, it is not recorded that he took an active part in the cultivation of his extensive gardens.

He encouraged wine-making in England, and perhaps he experimented with his own grapes in Hampshire.[15] Raymond Bush writes of a profitable vineyard planted by Lord Bute in Glamorganshire: "The vintage of 1881 was excellent in quality. Dr. Lawson Tait, late of Birmingham, a noted connoisseur of wines, bought several dozens of it."[16] Good wines and excellent cigars were an important part of his life-style; like Churchill, he was seldom seen without a cigar, as he drove to his hospital or relaxed after dinner.

Tait's choice of the New Forest for his country house was probably made to put him within nearer reach of London. In addition, for some years he held an appointment to a private hospital in Southampton. Here he operated quite frequently, for which activity he incurred much criticism.

About 1889 a small hospital in Southampton was established in a private house with (initially) only two beds. This was the Women's Free Hospital with a medical officer in charge, assisted by Lawson Tait as Consultant Surgeon and Dr. Playfair of London as Consultant Physician. Tait founded this hospital in the belief that no surgeon in the area was capable of doing the abdominal operations in which he specialised. Dr. E. F. Eliot, who had worked in Birmingham, was the medical officer; Tait trained him as his assistant and helped him with the difficult cases. The Southampton practitioners, understandably, did not approve of this invasion of their territory and questioned the ability of Eliot. They pointed out that the results of the operations performed were not reported and that Tait was usually in Birmingham rather than Southampton. The local Southampton Medical Society pressed for an enquiry. Tait repudiated all these criticisms and suggested that there was jealousy over Eliot's success, that there were many examples of consultants appointed to hospitals far from their home base and that in any case he had installed one of his most experienced nurses in the Southampton Hospital. The Consultant Physician, Dr. Playfair, resigned; however, Tait continued to visit the hospital sporadically until 1895. The *Lancet* was rather terse about all this. There were hints that, far from being a free hospital, patients were charged fees, and that Tait was out for financial gain to the detriment of the local surgeons. It was not a very happy venture and although Tait may have been altruistic in founding the hospital, as he frequently suggested, his case was not very convincing.[17]

There was an added attraction in the South, for Tait owned a yacht which he moored in the Solent. He does not appear to have ventured very far out, using it only for short cruises, and he delighted in entertaining his friends on board for picnics and dinner parties.

For a while, Tait owned a thatched cottage at Kings Bromley, which was rather more conveniently placed for short respites from Birminghham, as he loved to be in the country. He also had for a time a house in Cropthorne, with a houseboat on the Avon. He enjoyed taking his friends on the river and invariably cooked the meals himself, his repertoire being rather limited to the frying pan.

Tait was very fond of animals, particularly his beloved Persian cats, which he had in all his establishments. He was strongly opposed to blood sports, a feeling which undoubtedly influenced his support of the anti-vivisection movement.

For a man so intensely involved in an exacting profession it is almost unbelievable that there should have been time for so many unrelated activities and interests. His medical reading and writing must have taken up many of his spare hours. Yet he was well acquainted with general literature, drama, art, music, philosophy, archaeology and history. He retained a love of Scottish writers and could quote from Robert Burns at great length. He had strong views about Shakespeare (which he had first expressed publicly in Wakefield), believing that his plays "held the very heights and depths of human thought." He supported the theory that Francis Bacon had written some of the plays attributed to Shakespeare. He also collected old books in an erratic fashion.

There is some uncertainty about Tait's religious beliefs. It has been noted that he was most probably brought up in the Roman Catholic faith, but the evidence is uncertain. McKay made many attempts to find out his real feelings and concluded that Tait adhered to Unitarian principles and was not an atheist. Both McKay and Martin record long conversations with Tait on moral philosophy and on primitive religions; they found him extraordinarily well-informed on such subjects. Of the Roman Catholic Church he said: "That religion was a hard one to live up to, but an easy one to die in". He was fond of quoting Samuel Johnson's remark that "no rational man can die without uneasy apprehension." He pondered much on the question of immortality. McKay records that when Tait was in Rome in 1890 he had an audience with the Pope, who consulted him on the question: "Should the life of a foetus be considered before the life of the mother?".

There is an extant sermon which Tait preached in Birmingham in 1877. It was entitled "The Image of Baal". In his sermon Tait deplored the literal translation and acceptance of Biblical writings, considering this to be the cause of numerous sectarian differences in the Christian Church. He had stern criticisms to make of his Scottish countrymen brought up in the Calvinistic doctrine of pre-ordained election to, or exclusion from, eternal life, he said of Calvinism that "as I grew to man's estate I found this impressed upon the habits and thoughts of all around me." He had obviously rebelled:[18]

> I naturally reasoned that if I were one of the elect there could be no inducement for me to regard the precepts of Christ, when my inclination led me in another direction. On the converse, if I should not be in the favoured list, there was a similar absence of inducement for obedience to the moral law. To me a God who could make such a profitless bargain could not occupy the Temple; and therefore I put away the image of Baal which my fathers had made.

There follows a revealing passage in which Tait admitted that his ideas on religion were greatly influenced by his study of Darwin's evolutionary theory. He saw a possibility that Darwinism, as applied to physical life and structure, could present a better understanding of the moral nature of man. He deviates in his sermon to thoughts on ancestor worship, sun worship and Scandinavian mythology. He makes a scathing attack on orthodox Christian practice. He scorned those who declared in the Creed that they accepted "Father Almighty, Maker and Ruler of all things . . . in whose sight all men are equal", but who, he averred, really believed "that He favours some of His children to the detriment of others . . . that He is to be hoodwinked by lists of subscriptions and the wearing of phylacteries." He denounced those "who regard Him as the parish deity of Great Britain and pray Him not to go near the parish of Russia or France or America, or whatever spot of the earth's little surface happens to be at the time most hateful to us. . . ."

He ends with an appeal to understand a God of the Universe and with the belief than "an abandonment of the popular conception of God as a mere anthropomorphism would over the ages bring a purer and higher conception of a Godhead."

This sermon brings out Tait's Unitarian beliefs and his distaste for hypocrisy or cant. If it reads confusedly in places it does show his deep thinking and a degree of learning.

Tait was fascinated by the early history of the Christian Church and by primitive religions. He astonished McKay by expounding eruditely on phallic worship. He believed that the Tau (or T-shaped cross) of the

Crucifixion was adapted to Christian symbolism from the earlier Greek phallic symbol. The origins of words and symbols intrigued him greatly and he often surprised his friends by his etymological knowledge.

Whether in his antiquarian research or in his observation of the contemporary scene, Tait was always ready to apply some detail to his work. While travelling in a carriage he noticed in the coat of arms of the railway company a device of a complicated knot. He found out that it was part of the crest of the Stafford family and that the knot had been devised to hang criminals. He thought it must have been a very reliable knot; he tried it out and then applied it to ligate large pedicles otherwise difficult to secure during his operations. Thus was born the "Staffordshire knot" which Tait popularised and which he regarded as the safest surgical knot ever invented.

In 1876 Tait was elected to the Birmingham City Council, where he played an active part in local affairs. He served as Chairman of the Health Committee for some years. There were many local societies in which he participated, such as the Philosophical Society and the Birmingham Natural History Society, of which he was President. Somehow he found time to teach anatomy in the School of Art.

Tait had much to do with the affairs of Birmingham University. He was for a time Principal of Mason College. In 1887 he was appointed Professor of Gynaecology, and with his strong convictions about medical teaching he played a dominant part in shaping the Birmingham Medical School. Needless to say, this involved him in much argument and personal quarrels with his colleagues.

It is perhaps not surprising that, like some of his medical contemporaries, Tait could not resist entering a wider political arena. Soon after coming to Birmingham, by his contacts with George Dawson, he developed strong Liberal views. By 1886 he had become well known in political circles, numbering amongst his friends Sir William Harcourt, who lived near Tait in Hampshire and was a member of Gladstone's Cabinet.

In 1886 Gladstone and his government failed to push through a Bill in favour of Home Rule for Ireland, with the result that Parliament was dissolved on June 17th. The run-up to a General Election was remarkably short, Irish Home Rule being the only major issue. The Liberals had split and in Birmingham the majority were against Gladstone. Lawson Tait was firmly in support of Home Rule, and had already been active in advocating Irish independence. There was some confusion in the ranks of the Liberals, with the result that the Bordesley Division of Birmingham was at first without a Gladstonian candidate. Mr. Jesse

Collings stood as a Liberal–Unionist and after much rumor, Lawson Tait issued (on June 28th) an election manifesto.[19] One might have expected some original statements in this, but it was confined to a short paragraph referring only to the Home Rule question.

Tait held his first meeting on the same date. He denounced Collings as leaning over to the Conservatives. He had not much time to work up a following and was perhaps a bit half-hearted, for he said that "I must say that I came forward with no desire to possess a parliamentary distinction and nothing but the strongest emergency of the present situation would have induced me to become a candidate." It was a little unfortunate that he had to announce that his membership in the Liberal Party had lapsed! He held a meeting every night until voting took place and he answered his hecklers with good humour. Mr. Collings was a much more experienced politician, and perhaps it was not surprising that when the results were announced on July 5th Collings had received 4,475 votes and Tait only 1,040. Apart from Tait's inexperience it must be noted that Birmingham in general was strongly opposed to Irish Home Rule.

So ended a rather ill-prepared political venture. There was another election the following year, and Tait was expected to participate actively. A cartoon in a local satirical journal showed him sparring with Randolph Churchill, but Tait declined to be nominated again. Perhaps it was rather a pity that he did not enter the Commons, for he might have livened up the proceedings of the House and he could well have fought for medical and social causes with vigour and success.

In the field of medico-politics it was unlikely that he should have failed to make some mark, but he met with much opposition in his efforts to gain any position of real power. In the Edinburgh College of Surgeons he did not seek office on a Council which was at the time parochial in its influence. There are indications that he did have some interest, for there is in the College an oil painting of the Council and Fellows of 1891 in which Tait is clearly portrayed.[20]

Tait recognised that surgical influence was in the hands of the English College of which he had become both Member and Fellow. He was a frequent critic of the College, deploring its domination by London surgeons and by a group largely confined to a select few of the teaching hospitals. He strongly supported the principle that provincial surgeons should have more effective voting rights and greater representation on the Council. He also favoured the view that Members of the College should have some say in its management, being Vice-President of their own association. He belonged to an active Association of Fellows who sought to overthrow London's domination. On such platforms he offered himself as a candidate in the Council Election of 1889. As was customary, he wrote to the medical press expressing his views and deploring the fact that provincial Fellows could have only a proxy vote. He was unsuccessful; he polled only 177 votes and the three vacancies were filled by well-established London surgeons. He stood again in 1890; on this occasion he was joined by another candidate from the Provinces, William Mitchell Banks (1842-1904) of Liverpool. The *Lancet* was favourable to the idea of provincial representation and said of Tait that "No Fellow is more fitted to fight boldly for the provincials and for thoroughgoing reform." Although Tait did rather better this second time, he was not elected. Mitchell Banks headed the list over two London surgeons. Tait stood once more in 1891, but was again unsuccessful. On the whole, he took his defeats with dignity but he did protest that Banks' supporters had been advised not to cast a second vote for Tait. Although he had originally announced that he would go on standing for the Council until he was successful, he refused nomination in 1892 and never entered the lists again. Perhaps his chances were poor since he had attacked the College so vehemently. Over one particular quarrel he had threatened to bring a litigation against Sir William Savory, the President.

In February 1889 the Association of College Members arranged for a meeting to be held within the College to discuss reform and did not, as the laws demanded, seek permission from the Council. The College was closed on the appointed day, and two members brought an action against the President. Lawson Tait joined the fray and brought his own action to the tune of £2,500! The members' case was brought to trial in the Chancery Division of the High Court in 1892 and was dismissed. Meanwhile Tait's case was held in abeyance, and we presume he sensibly withdrew it. This kind of thing made it unlikely that the London surgeons would support him and that there would not have been any help from those such as Spencer Wells, an influential past-President. It may be, however, that much needed reforms which came eventually were hastened by Tait's constant criticisms.[21]

In his own specialty Tait exerted considerable influence by his involvement in a new organisation – the British Gynaecological Society. In 1884 a group of gynaecologists from all over the country met under the chairmanship of Dr. Routh and established the Society.[22] Dissatisfaction was expressed that gynaecology was linked so closely with obstetrics. The London Obstetrical Society was criticised for failing to give a fair share of time to gynaecological contributions. Most of all the gynaecologists wished to "establish firmly the right to carry out surgical treament of our own cases." The curious situation prevailed by which a practitioner appointed to a hospital as an obstetrician or physician-accoucheur (and often developing a predominant interest in gynaecology) was debarred from doing abdominal operations on his own cases. This rule was particularly common in the London teaching hospitals. With the increasing exploitation of abdominal section in the diagnosis and management of diseases of the uterus and its appendages (due very largely to Tait's teaching), this veto was becoming quite intolerable. Although the Society was primarily interested in establishing gynaecology as a specialty in its own right, it does seem that it represented yet another move to bring the provincials into equality with London surgeons in their activities and influence. The first president to be elected was Dr. Alfred Meadows (1833-1887) of St. Mary's Hospital. Four other London surgeons and Lawson Tait were elected as Vice-Presidents. Tait was not at the inaugural meeting, but a letter giving his full support was read. He was to be one of the most active participants in the new Society.

Meadows gave his presidential address at the first full meeting in 1885, stressing once more the objects of the Society, not least of which was the importance of participation by those outside of London.[23] He expressed the hope "that giant Lawson Tait" would contribute and that on occasion the Society would travel to Birmingham or other centres outside London for their meetings. He announced that there would be full reports in a journal published by the Society.

Tait at once became a frequent contributer to the Society in its monthly meetings, delivering papers, showing specimens and always joining in the discussions. He succeeded Dr. Meadows as President; in his inaugural address "On some pending questions in Gynaecology," given in January 1887, he announced that there were already 460 members. He discussed the more notable papers given since the start of the Society and devoted a lot of time to comments on the Imlach case in Liverpool (a matter to which reference is made later). He could not resist the opportunity of attacking Spencer Wells once more. (Spencer Wells and some other distinguished London gynaecologists did not join this Society).

Tait was very proud to be the first provincial President of a society which met in London. He wound up his year of office with an address on the "Work and progress of the British Gynaecological Society". Once more he got into medico-politics, attacking in particular, the *Lancet*, which for some reason refused to report the proceedings of the Society. Granville Bantock succeeded as President and Tait continued to give a profusion of papers, all of which were published in the Society's journal. In 1890 he attended no meetings, partly because of poor health. In 1891 he attended on at least twenty occasions, but thereafter his name appears infrequently in the reports.

It is difficult to estimate the influence which this Society exerted on gynaecology in Great Britain. Today Obstetrics and Gynaecology remain together under the influence of a joint Royal College. Tait would have been pleased to know that in 1929 the first President of the Royal College of Obstetricians and Gynaecologists was a provincial, William Blair-Bell (1871-1936) of Liverpool. If the British Gynaecological Society, which disbanded in 1907 to join with the Obstetrical Society of London to form a section of the Royal Society of Medicine, did not succeed in making gynaecology a specialty on its own it certainly had beneficial influences. In the early years Tait had much to do with its success, this being one of his more successful ventures into the London scene.

It must be admitted that through his participation in the activities of so many medical societies, Tait was mainly intent on finding platforms from which he could preach his own dogmatic ideas and enter into warfare with his antagonists. His numerous contributions to the annual meetings of the British Medical Association and to the Midlands Branch of the Association have been indicated. Although he was the president of the local association, he was never in the hierarchy of the Association. In general he supported it but there were occasions when he threatened to resign as a result of arguments concerning the administration. Locally he was a prominent member of the Birmingham Medical Institute, of which he became President in 1889. Some of his most important papers were first given to this Society.

Lawson Tait was an enthusiastic traveller. For some of his contemporaries, like Spencer Wells, foreign travel was a recreation; to Tait it was an opportunity to impress his personality and ideas on foreign colleagues. He seldom went abroad for pleasure but rather for consultations or, as with his visit to the United States, to participate in surgical meetings. When he had some professional excuse to travel he invariably viewed anything of interest, found out all he could about each country and added to his collection of antiques and curios. There were many trips to Europe. He visited Italy several times, on one occasion to recuperate from an illness but usually to consult or operate.

By 1880 Lawson Tait's work and reputation were well known in the United States. His books and other writings had attracted much attention and many American gynaecologists who visited Great Britain went straight to Birmingham to see his work, some remaining for several months as his pupils. In 1881 his friend Marion Sims wrote that "Lawson Tait has gone ahead of us all in opening up new diseases of abdominal surgery. . . . He is now the leader in this department of Surgery and has succeeded in opening up fields of great fertility which we may all freely cultivate with great profit."[24] In 1883 he was elected an Honorary Fellow of the American Gynaecological Society; the following year he received invitations to lecture and demonstrate his operative techniques from individuals such as Professor Vander Veer and from bodies such as the Canadian Medical Association.

His visit to Canada took place in the summer of 1884. From the account he gave later in a lecture to his Birmingham colleagues, and from reports in the medical press, we can piece together a tour which was in many respects triumphal. He sailed from Liverpool to Quebec, his arrival enlivened by an accident to a young lady passenger who cut her arm on a pane of glass. Tait was called in and, acquiring a few instruments and some chloroform, was successful in ligating a severed brachial artery.

Having gained a certain amount of publicity by his prompt and skilful action, Tait then set out on a hectic tour of North America. He lectured in Montreal on abdominal surgery, his views gaining general acceptance, although he was criticised for taking the opportunity to launch yet another personal attack on Spencer Wells, who was well thought of in North America.[25] He went on to Boston where he was delighted to view the sponge used by Morton when he administered the first ether anaesthetic for a surgical operation. He was intrigued at seeing the skeleton of John Collins Warren (1778-1856), the surgeon who performed this historic operation in 1846. Warren was one of the most distinguished American surgeons of the early nineteenth century; on his death, his will directed that his skeleton be carefully preserved and mounted for the edification of future generations. Tait wrote of his own macabre satisfaction in shaking the hand of the grisly remains: "a hand the bony elements of which I had the privilege of touching, for with a great conceit he now himself forms part of his own museum".[26]

He visited Philadelphia, Washington and New York. He was greatly impressed with the Women's Medical College in Philadelphia and with the Medical Library in Washington. He found surgeons in all these centres more receptive to his ideas than were his British colleagues, feeling perhaps that his ability and authority were at long last gaining proper recognition. He thought Americans were stimulating; he admired their institutions and their readiness to travel abroad. Most of all, he appreciated their support of his views.

In his memoir of Lawson Tait, written in 1899, Charles Reed comments on suggestions that Tait was to some degree critical of American surgeons.[27] He had at times been offended at the numerous American visitors to England who "ran up to Birmingham for a day just to see him operate," and then went off without having bothered to know him or to have understood his methods. He had publicly described such visitors as "tramps." Reed visited Tait in 1886 and dined with him in Birmingham. When asked about his true attitude Tait replied: "No, far from disliking Americans I am really very fond of them. I owe them a debt of gratitude that I cannot easily repay; if it had not been for the recognition and support they gave me, and are yet giving me, I could not have succeeded in my fight against English conservatism".

He was honoured by the Americans more than he was by his own countrymen. In addition to honorary membership in several societies, he was awarded the L.L.D. degree from two universities.[28] In 1887 he was elected a Vice-president of the International Congress which met in Washington, but he did not attend this meeting. He was made an Honorary Consulting Surgeon to the Brooklyn Hospital, where he had operated on his visit in 1884.

At an early stage in his professional career Lawson Tait became aware of many injustices inflicted on his fellow practitioners. Litigation against doctors was frequent and in many cases a doctor quite innocent of malpractice could emerge unscathed only if he was able to meet heavy legal expenses. Then too, despite the Medical Act of 1857, the profession (and the public) were ill-protected against quacks and illegal practitioners. Doctors often depended on financial assistance from their colleagues to save themselves from bankruptcy after some legal action. Friends generally rallied to help if a case was unfairly judged, and the name of Lawson Tait often appeared generously in lists of subscribers. In the eighties there were some notable cases which brought to a head the question of the desirability of creating an organisation for the protection of the doctor. The Bradley case in 1884 was an example. Dr. Bradley was convicted, on sparse evidence, of a criminal assault on a woman patient and served eight months of a sentence of hard labour before he was given a free pardon by the Home Secretary. Tait was prominent amongst those who assisted him financially and pressed for his release.[29]

A Medical Defence Association had been established in 1875, but it was not actively supported by the profession with the result that its effectiveness was hampered by lack of funds. In 1885 the Medical Defence Union was founded by a group of laymen, the prime mover being the secretary, a Mr. Rideal. The Union sought to link itself with the British Medical Association, but this offer was rejected on the grounds of "dangerous pecuniary responsibility." The need for a more powerful organisation was pressed, and medical support gathered rapidly. Local branches were established, including one in Birmingham in 1886. Lawson Tait accepted the notion that a powerful Defence Union was something badly needed by the profession. He chaired the first meeting of the Birmingham branch, was elected as the local President, and became President of the national organisation the following year. He threw himself into its work with his usual vigour and soon there were more than five hundred members. There was criticism at first, for only in a few rather trivial cases had any doctors been helped. The *Lancet,* in particular, was lukewarm about its activities. However, after a shaky start, thanks to Tait's drive, the Union became well established and effective. Unfortunately, there was trouble with the Secretary, Mr. Rideal, over his salary. Tait initiated a litigation against Rideal for the return of part of the salary paid to him. The matter was settled, but not without some difficulty. In time, the organisation became solvent and Tait forecast its increasing success. The *British Medical Journal* was less optimistic and offered its opinion that "Mr. Lawson Tait has taken on his shoulders, unwisely we fear, a heavy responsibility and a thankless task." But this was just the kind of challenge in which Tait revelled. He continued as President while Rideal, who deserves applause for launching the scheme, retired into obscurity. In 1888 Tait moved the headquarters to Birmingham, where it came to be dominated by provincial instead of London doctors. At an early stage the Union challenged the General Medical Council, particularly with regard to its judicial procedures against doctors, but it was to be another seventy-five years before reform was achieved. Until 1893 Tait managed the affairs of the Union ably and, at first, with the acceptance of the profession. Antagonism grew towards him, one member stating wryly that "Tait *is* the Medical Defence Union, supported by puppets." The question arose as to whether or not the Union should intervene in quarrels between members of the profession and Tait was himself involved in a test case. Three years previously the Royal College of Surgeons had threatened to deprive him of the privileges of membership and fellowship because he had contravened a byelaw in supporting the calling of a meeting of the Association of Members without permission of the College Council. As has already been noted, Tait tried to bring an action against the President of the College, persuading the Union to support him. There was criticism over the payment of some of the costs to Tait by the Union, especially since he had promised to refund any such payments.

A more serious cause of antagonism to Tait was over the Denholm case which, as will be described in the next chapter, had other repercussions. This was an episode in which Tait was directly involved; again he recouped some of his costs from the Medical Defence Union. The *British Medical Journal* commented that "it would have been more desirable in view of Tait's social and professional position for the costs to have come from his own pocket than from the coffers of a young and struggling Association." Almost inevitably Tait offered his resignation, admitting that "my Presidency brings trouble in the Union which another man might avoid"; but he maintained that he had acted correctly. Some of the attacks upon him undoubtedly came from London practitioners who did not think that a provincial should have been allowed to dominate the Union for so long. Victor Horsley succeeded Tait as President and restored and increased the confidence of the profession. The Medical Defence Union still survives as an indispensable organisation for the protection of doctors and some of the credit for its establishment must be given to Lawson Tait.[30]

Although he had done some experimental work on animals as a student and in his early years in Birmingham, Tait soon took up a firm stance against vivisection. His attitudes were influenced by an intense love of animals and an antipathy for blood sports. His arguments were based on his belief that the results of animal experiments could not be applied to man.

The events leading up to the bitter quarrels concerning animal experimentation may be traced briefly. Before 1871 there was a relatively uncritical acceptance of the use of animals in medical research, but in that year the physiologists, Sanderson and Foster, published a *Handbook to the Physiological Laboratory.* This created much criticism for its detailed descriptions of animal experiments. A public outcry developed, often hysterical in nature, and forced the establishment of a Royal Commission, which issued its report in 1876. Although the English physiologists were acquitted of abuse, a Bill was presented in

Parliament to place the responsibility for the control of animal laboratorities in the hands of the Home Secretary. The comment was made that, in its original form, this Bill "acquitted the accused and sentenced them to be under the surveillance of the police for life." A cartoon in *Punch* depicted a censorious policeman pointing an accusing finger at a group of eminent doctors engaged in an experiment on a frog. Recognisable in the group are the leading champions in favour of animal experimentation – Sir William Jenner, Sir James Paget, Sir William Gull, and Dr. Ernest Hart. The caption reads: "*Operating Professor:* 'By this experiment we have ascertained that we can alleviate the sufferings of thousands of our fellow countrymen. . . .' *Policeman interrupting:* 'No you mayn't. We've had enough o' this sort of thing, you must move on'. *Professor:* 'Move on, we can't *move* if *you* interfere'." Professional opposition to the Bill, initiated largely by Ernest Hart, resulted later in a Vivisection Act which was amended in such a way as to make it more acceptable to the doctors. In 1882, the public outcry having lost none of its force, another Bill was presented for the abolition of animal experiments; this, however, failed completely.

Around 1880 feeling ran particularly high over animal experimentation and the controversy was acute in Birmingham. Sampson Gamgee (1828-1886), a Birmingham surgeon, published a pamphlet entitled "Vivisection and Human Surgery", in which he affirmed that animal experimentation was essential for the development of medicine and surgery. In a debate at the Birmingham Philosophical Society, Tait led the opposition to Gamgee with a paper entitled "The Uselessness of experiments on animals as an Instrument in Scientific research".[31] Tait saw no justification for repeating the many standard animal experiments used to instruct the student; he attacked blood sports; he argued that animals had equal rights with humans. Most of all, however, he denied that anything useful had been learnt concerning the actions of drugs in human disease by animal experiment. He attempted to show that the most important advances in surgery had been made by practical clinicians who were uninfluenced by experimental work. Most of the audience were against Tait's views, certainly the doctors. His case was not helped by the presence of some rather hysterical ladies who were on his side.

On the whole, Tait did not come out very well in this debate, but he continued to fight ardently against vivisection. He wrote a letter to the *British Medical Journal* offering a prize of £500 for an essay proving the benefits of vivisection and indicated that if such an essay were convincing he would withdraw what he had said at the Birmingham discussion. No record has been found to suggest that anyone put in an essay for this prize, which is surprising, considering the size of the award![32]

Tait's interventions were not always consistent. He is said to have modified his views and allowed that bacteriological research using animals was permissible and necessary to medical progress. This admission was often used against him by those in favour of vivisection.

In 1892 there was a notable debate on vivisection at the Church Congress under the chairmanship of the Archbishop of Canterbury.[33] At the start of the meeting it was asked why Lawson Tait, accepted as a prominent anti-vivisectionist, was not present. The reply was that Tait was not eligible to attend as he was not a "convinced Churchman." Amongst other notable doctors Victor Horsley spoke in favour of animal experimentation, stating that Lawson Tait was the only doctor of any status opposed to it; Horsley did admit to Tait's skill as a surgeon, but claimed that he was not a scientist. A leader in the *British Medical Journal* dealt harshly with Tait, particularly as he had not participated in the many discussions which had taken place at Association meetings. He was also criticised for a letter to the *Times* in which he had challenged his medical colleagues with "strange witlessness and lack of good taste."[34]

Later in 1892 Tait attended in London a well publicised meeting of the Anti-Vivisection Society. He was introduced by an ardent clerical opponent of vivisection, Canon Wilberforce, as "that eminent physiologist of whom it is said that he is reckoned as the most skilful operator in Europe."[35] Tait spoke at length, rather unscientifically and rather emotionally. He announced, "I regret that I have to offer to the British Public an apology on behalf of my profession and I do so with a sense of degradation. . . ." He stated that he had been prohibited from attending the Church Congress, but admitted that there were circumstances in his history which rendered it a doubtful matter as to whether he was a member of the Church of England! His utterances aroused considerable anger, not least his apology to the British Public. Some thought he ought to resign from the British Medical Association. There followed a weary correspondence in the medical journals, and it may be generally said that Tait's position with regard to vivisection now appeared to be somewhat equivocal. Nonetheless, the anti-vivisectionists regarded him as one of their most important medical protagonists. Over many years he attacked various individuals who had used animal experimentation in their research. Even James Syme did not escape, but he had died long before and was past caring. In an argument over the sensitivity of the peritoneum to pain, Tait was easily routed by Charles Sherrington. All in all his intervention in this controversy probably harmed his reputation in many quarters.

It is interesting to record that these activities were echoed many years later when in 1959 a group of opponents of animal experimentation founded a Lawson Tait Research Trust "to encourage the development of methods of research which although not using experiments on living animals nevertheless produce results which significantly affect medical progress." Tait's name was attached as a memorial to him as "Father and Perfector of Abdominal Surgery" as well as for his battle against vivisection.[36]

In the years leading up to 1892, which proved to be a sad turning point in Tait's life, there were fewer original contributions to gynaecology and surgery from him than in earlier years. His writings were as frequent as ever and he never missed an opportunity to give papers to societies or to participate in discussions. Mostly Tait now drove home the lessons he had already attempted to teach—his insistence on abdominal section for diagnosis of doubtful cases, his advocacy of urgent operation for acute conditions, and justification of his operation to remove chronically inflamed appendages. He was becoming rather less certain of the value of removing appendages for fibroids of the uterus, and he had come to accept the desirability of more frequent recourse to local excision of a tumour or to a hysterectomy. In his continued advocacy of removal of the appendages for chronic inflammatory disease he still had to fight the battle against those who described such operations as "spaying", those who suggested that he was advocating wholesale sterilisation of women (forgetting, as they did, that the diseases concerned had made these women sterile already) and those who maintained, on rather uncertain evidence, that his operations had deleterious effects on the sexual life of his patients. Tait found it difficult to demolish these moral and ethical arguments, despite the fact that they were generally ill-founded and also much exaggerated.

The arguments over the "spaying operation" reached a peak over an affair in Liverpool concerning a local surgeon, Francis Imlach (1851-1920).[37] Imlach was an Edinburgh graduate who had settled in Liverpool and rapidly established himself as a progressive and versatile surgeon who had been influenced by Tait's teaching. He (Imlach) was also largely instrumental in founding the new Liverpool Women's Hospital in 1883, to which he was appointed a surgeon. The senior surgeon was Dr. Thomas Grimsdale (1823-1902), who was conservative in his outlook with regard to operative intervention for gynaecological conditions. Imlach presented various papers to the Liverpool Medical Institution between 1884 and 1885 in which he described many successful operations for severe inflammatory disease of the appendages. There was considerable criticism in the discussion of these papers, led by Grimsdale and the Professor of Midwifery, John Wallace (1839-1898), both of whom (along with others) viewed with concern the excessive frequency with which exploratory abdominal operations were being performed at the Women's Hospital.[38]

In 1885 Imlach operated on a young unmarried woman and removed, in consecutive operations, both ovaries which he found to be diseased and which he believed were the cause of her symptoms. Imlach suspected that she also had a renal calculus, especially when such symptoms persisted after the ovarian operations. The patient consulted Mr. Frank Paul (1851-1941), a young surgeon who was to achieve considerable fame. Dr. William Carter presented her case at the local medical society in February of 1886.[39] He brought it forward "from a sense of duty and painful responsibility." He claimed that the removal of the ovaries had been unwarranted, that the patient had been unsexed and that no explanation to either the patient or to her husband had been made before the operations. After the patient consulted Frank Paul the latter removed the large renal stone and subsequently did a successful removal of the infected kidney.

Quite clearly this was a general attack on the whole conception of aggressive surgery for gynaecological conditions based on the fear, at times justifiable, that unnecessary operations were being performed. Behind it all, however, it is all too likely that this was a vicious personal attack on Francis Imlach. Whether this arose from jealousy at his undoubted successes, perhaps to the detriment of the private practice of his conservative seniors, or whether there were other personal reasons is uncertain. Imlach was present at the meeting. He had already refuted the general charges of over-operating in discussions following his papers in the previous year. He had quoted his own figures of 128 operations for pathological conditions of the appendages with a mortality of 6.2 per cent, against Professor Wallace's meagre statistics of twelve operations with a 50 per cent mortality. Imlach stated positively that in the case under discussion the ovaries were diseased.

Quite without warning Dr. Grimsdale seized the opportunity to propose a motion to set up an enquiry into the "practice and ethics of these operations" in the Women's Hospital. A Committee of Enquiry was elected, with Grimsdale himself nominating the members. Although the brief was to investigate the operative work done at the Women's Hospital, it was very obvious that this was an enquiry into Imlach's surgical activities in general. Eight months later a report, awaited with some excitement both locally and nationally, was produced.[40]

Meanwhile, the unfortunate Imlach found himself involved in litigation over another case, which came before the Assizes in August 1886. Imlach had operated on a married woman, one Mrs. Casey, and had removed the ovary and tube which were involved by a chronic swelling caused by a previous haemorrhage. The plaintiff's case was that the operation was unnecessary and was done without consent of the patient and without explanation to her or to the husband. In addition it was claimed that there had been no consultation with any other surgeon (as required by the rules of the hospital) and that the patient had been "unsexed". Counsel for the plaintiff regarded the charge as one of negligence and brought a large group of witnesses to support his charge.

It was inevitable that the witnesses for the plaintiff included Wallace and Grimsdale, who were not only conservative in their attitudes to surgical intervention but were also opposed to Imlach personally. The only point which they could make was that Imlach had failed to obey the rules of the hospital by not seeking a second opinion before operating. In his defence, Imlach insisted that the operation was necessary and stated that he had explained the operation to his patient. He was supported by experts whose authority carried much more weight than that of the local doctors. Lawson Tait was called and said that the operation was "most proper"; he did not hesitate to criticise Grimsdale as "out of date." He was followed in turn by accepted experts—Aveling, Savage and Greig Smith—and by Dr. Marsh, a local general practitioner. Finally a nurse from the hospital confirmed that the patient had been told about the consequences of the operation. The jury had no hesitation in clearing Imlach's name with costs to the plaintiff.

The trial and the instigation of the Medical Institution Enquiry created considerable local excitement. There was a spate of letters to the local press from both supporters and opponents of Imlach. Many letters—the more virulent—were anonymous; many came from the clergy and patients either satisfied or dissatisfied with Imlach's treatment. The general trend was to suggest that some surgeons were ruthlessly unsexing the poor women of Liverpool and exposing them to experimentation. Many of the subscribers to the Women's Hospital threatened to withdraw their support. It was suggested by one correspondent that Lawson Tait had intervened officiously and rudely. He wrote several angry letters to the *Liverpool Courier.* The first was in criticism of a letter by Spencer Wells in which the latter had replied to an enquiry from the secretary of the Women's Hospital. Wells had been asked for his confidential opinion about the frequency with which abdominal operations had been performed in Liverpool; he had replied briefly that the rate was "so shocking as to be almost incredible." Wells' letter should not have been published, and Tait at once wrote to say that he too had been asked for his private opinion but that this had rightly remained confidential. He pointed out that the statistics of the Samaritan Hospital in London, where Wells worked, revealed an identical percentage of cases submitted to abdominal section. Tait was then attacked in the local press for daring to contradict Wells, and more than one correspondent suggested that Tait's opinion was worthless. The latter did not take this lying down; he insisted that his opinions were recognised as being as authoritative as those of Wells. Finally, he accused Grimsdale of having encouraged Mrs. Casey to bring an action against Imlach.

In this heated atmosphere the Medical Institution Committee brought out their report. It was a reasoned document with no personal attack on Imlach but clearly against him, since he had done the majority of the operations scrutinised by the Committee. Two recommendations were made: that no operation should be done without a second opinion, except in a real emergency, and that patients should be given a clear explanation before any operation. An official for the Women's Hospital was privately instructed to persuade Imlach to accept these rules. It seems that he refused to agree to the recommendation about consultation; if he was obstinate about this it was partly because of his character and partly because he was opposed to rules which prevented the obstetrician or gynaecologist from doing abdominal procedures.

Not surprisingly, the Hospital authorities were greatly alarmed at the adverse publicity caused by Imlach's trial and by the Enquiry. At the annual meeting of the Liverpool Women's Hospital in 1887 Imlach came up for re-election only to be rejected after a somewhat suspect organisation of proxy votes.

This chain of events undoubtedly ruined Imlach's promising career. He had to retire from consultant practice and despite a constant battle he was never reinstated. Many of his colleagues supported him, and a long battle was waged in the Medical Institution. Imlach himself claimed that he had been victimised and that Grimsdale had rigged the composition of the Enquiry Committee against him. Many members of the Institution considered that the Enquiry was unconstitutional and that the report should be deleted from the Minutes. There was, in fact, a rule that ethical matters should not be discussed in the Institution; it was obvious that this rule had been broken. An attempt in 1887 to overthrow the Enquiry was unsuccessful, but feelings in support of Imlach were demonstrated by the presentation to him of a testimonial in the form of £600 from his colleagues. In 1900 another attempt was made to withdraw the Institution Enquiry under the leadership of Robert Jones, Thomas Bickerton and James Barr, but this too was unsuccessful. Long after Imlach's death Dr. C.G. Hughes wrote a rather touching letter to the Institution in a belated effort to make some amends to Imlach. He made only the modest request that Imlach's portrait, if presented to the Institution, should be hung there for posterity. The request was granted, but this was no more than a feeble recognition of the injustice inflicted on a young pioneer who, like Lawson Tait, fought to introduce new and necessary surgical advances but who fell instead into a reprehensible attack waged against him by jealous colleagues.

Tait saw the Imlach case as part of his own battle against conservatism in surgery. As well as playing an important role in Imlach's trial, he conducted a long campaign in support of Imlach against those who opposed him, never sparing their reputations. On the whole, the medical journals supported Imlach, admitting the danger of excessive enthusiasm for radical gynaecological operations, but accepting the need for surgical advance and the validity of the new operations which Tait had developed. It does seem that the Liverpool episode did something to clear the air and that it led to a more reasoned acceptance of the new gynaecology. Despite considerable local criticism of Tait's interventions in the Imlach case, in some quarters his help must have been recognised, for he was appointed an Honorary Surgeon to the Women's Hospital.[41]

Between 1880 and 1890 there was a wave of enthusiasm for the treatment of simple uterine tumours by electricity. This had been introduced by Georges Apostoli (1847-1900), who believed that bleeding was controlled and that tumours might regress if submitted to the galvanic current by use of suitably placed electrodes. Tait attacked any clinician who employed this method. There was good reason to do so, for many used "electrolysis" without much precision in diagnosis and without very careful documentation of their results. Tait wrote: "I condemn the whole thing because it is becoming a fertile field for quackery, the lamentable tale of every attempt to apply the electrical current for the relief of human suffering". Tait did take the trouble to go to Paris to see Apostoli's work, but he was not impressed. He did buy a battery and use the treatment on his own patients without success. In 1891 he wrote that "my operating rooms are now being flooded with a collection of failures of electrical treatment." (It was his unguarded criticism of the application of electrical treatment in a particular case which, as we shall see, contributed towards his downfall in 1892.) When it was suggested that electricity should also be used to arrest the development of an extra-uterine pregnancy Tait was even more vociferous in his condemnations, describing the idea as "the most nonsensical proposal ever submitted to a surgical audience." James Aveling had proposed in 1886 that an early tubal pregnancy could be punctured with an electrode and destroyed by an electric current. Tait pointed out that it was nearly impossible to diagnose an early tubal pregnancy until it ruptured and caused either generalised acute bleeding or a local swelling in the region of the tube. Others believed that the more rare advanced and surviving tubal pregnancy could be treated by electricity. Tait said that the foetus could survive only occasionally in such cases and he condemned those who "murdered the child." In his denunciation of electrical treatment for such conditions Tait was undoubtedly correct, and in due course the method fell into disrepute despite support from some of the more influential gynaecologists.

Although Tait did not continue to practise obstetrics after his early years in Birmingham, he saw many patients with late complications after childbirth and a few with acute and unusual crises during labour. He was inevitably interested in the operation of Caesarean section. This procedure had a long history but it remained a very dangerous operation to the mother. In a paper as late as 1890 Tait estimated the maternal mortality to be as high as ninety to ninety-five per cent. Such disastrous results were related to many factors. First of all, the operation was not usually done until the mother was exhausted by a long drawn out labour, impeded by pelvic obstruction or other causes. Secondly, many such operations were performed in patients' homes rather than in hospitals. Thirdly, in home deliveries the work was done by gen-

general practitioners or obstetricians with little surgical training. There was also a curious technical point, namely that for many years operators were reluctant to suture the wound in the uterus, depending instead on natural contraction of the organ to induce healing. As the operation was generally performed after prolonged manipulations which almost invariably would have infected the uterine cavity, it is not surprising that results were poor and indeed it was remarkable that any women survived at all. It was an index of the dissatisfaction of surgeons and obstetricians with Caesarean section that in 1876 the Italian Eduardo Porro (1842-1902) introduced a new operation. He suggested that immediately after extraction of the child a hysterectomy should be done. The technique he devised was to open the abdomen and do a Caesarean section, put an elastic ligature around the neck of the uterus, amputate it and exteriorise the stump. Porro's operation caught on rapidly and the mortality rate was very much less than that for Caesarean section. By 1890 R.P. Harris of Philadelphia collected 264 cases from Europe and America with a maternal mortality rate much lower than that for Caesarean section.[42]

Tait was attracted to this idea in 1884 when he heard a paper by Clement Godson who described a successful "Caesarean section followed by removal of the uterus."[43] By 1890 Tait had done seven such operations with only one death, admitting to his own limited but disastrous experience of three Caesarean sections, all of which died. In the same year he expanded on his views on this subject in a paper to the Southampton Medical Society, entitled "On the surgical aspects of impacted labour". He told his audience that his incursions into the field of obstetrics were rare but he nevertheless felt that he could with justification discuss the place of abdominal operations in the management of labour complications. He deplored the tendency on the part of practitioners to deliver the infant in a case of obstructed labour by the crude methods of cranial perforation or evisceration. He emphasised that as an alternative, Caesarean section was attended by an unaccepted mortality rate which, in his opinion, was due to sepsis in the retained uterus. He then advocated Porro's principle of hysterectomy after extraction of the child by abdominal section. On this and other occasions he made the "Porro-Caesarean" operation sound rather simple.

As an advocate of Porro's operation for obstructed labour caused by contraction of the pelvis, Tait further suggested that it should be used for severe bleeding in placenta praevia and that if done quickly, both mother and child might survive. It is not certain that he ever attempted this operation in such a situation, nor was the idea received very favourably by obstetricians. For a brief period the Porro procedure was considered to be an advance in obstetric surgery, some surgeons referring to it as the Tait-Porro operation. Soon after 1890, however, the technique of Caesarean section was greatly improved and the general acceptance of aseptic or antiseptic principles reduced the risks. Porro's operation almost completely disappeared except for rare cases of obstructed labour caused by tumours of the neck of the uterus.

In 1891 Tait made an original clinical observation in the field of gynaecological pathology for which he is not generally awarded any priority. He gave a paper to the Royal Medico-Chirurgical Society entitled "The association of pleural effusion with diseases of the abdomen". Most of the cases he described were examples of co-existing chest and abdominal effusions in advanced malignant disease. In one case, however, pleural effusions were tapped thirty times, after which Tait explored the abdomen to find a "fibroid tumour" of the ovary. This he removed, with the result that the chest effusions did not recur thereafter. The case conforms to that presently described as Meigs' syndrome, a rare type of fibroid tumour of the ovary with peritoneal and pleural effusions. J.V. Meigs, an American gynaecologist, elucidated the condition in 1937 in both its clinical and pathological aspects.[44] Meigs was aware of Tait's case and linked his name with that of a French Surgeon named Demons, who had described a similar cure in 1887. It must be admitted that Tait showed little interest in the pathological details of his case; when he published it he used it rather to stress once more the desirability of abdominal section in doubtful conditions. Nevertheless he deserves credit for an early description of the successful treatment of this curious disease.

Tait was now producing few new ideas with regard to general abdominal surgery. He continued his reports on gallbladder surgery, limited to the operation of cholecystostomy, and remained in the forefront in surgery of the kidney. We have already indicated that he rolled out his long series of abdominal sections, a performance surpassing that of any other surgeon of the time. Most of the lectures, articles and letters pertaining to such topics are larded with antagonism towards Listerism, criticism of those with different views and, regrettably, at times a public exposure of colleagues who, in Tait's opinion, had mismanaged particular cases. There was one particularly virulent argument with Spencer Wells about such a case and a blatant accusation of lack of diagnostic and operative skill.[45]

In 1889 Tait published the first volume of a new book entitled *Diseases of Women and Abdominal Surgery.* This was largely a recapitulation of his earlier works. It is unfortunate that the second volume, which presumably would have elaborated on his enormous experience of general conditions in the abdomen, never appeared. It is probable that his ill health about this time, as well as the subsequent crises in his professional life, prevented the completion of this work. He wrote in 1892, "Truly I found art long and life brief and struggle all I can, but time fails me to get out my second volume". He was still trying to complete the book in 1895.

It was written of Tait that "no great surgical position was ever made so rapidly nor lost with such pathetic suddenness" and that "the last years of his life closed with pitiable obscurity." He undoubtedly suffered an eclipse in 1892, which the loyal McKay attributes simply to poor health and a sensible desire to take life more slowly. The factors which contributed to his unhappy decline are the subject of the next chapter.

CHAPTER IX
DECLINE AND FALL

Around 1892 certain circumstances contributed to a rapid decline in Lawson Tait's position and influence. He had now been accepted in Great Britain, albeit grudgingly, as a pioneer and few could fail to accord him a reasonable degree of credit for his contributions to surgery. His reputation, as has been shown, was rather more generously conceded in North America. This is reflected by an incident which occurred when the American gynaecologist Dr. Franklin Martin of Chicago, an ardent disciple of Tait, visited London in 1895 on the occasion of the Annual Meeting of the British Medical Association. The British Gynaecological Society gave a banquet to celebrate the meeting; it was attended by many distinguished British and foreign surgeons. Martin found himself seated near Lister and Lawson Tait. He had not met Tait before and at once fell under his spell, even though Tait was rather brusque with him. There were many speeches and toasts to the distinguished visitors; in return, the American surgeon John B. Murphy proposed the health of Lister, which was accorded with acclamation. Martin, to his embarrassment—he considered himself a nonentity in such distinguished company—was also asked to speak:[1]

> First I paid my respects to the surgeons of England. . . then I said that it was a rare privilege to meet Lister and his able followers face to face. There was however one phase of surgical England that we from afar, probably because of our better perspective, were unable to comprehend, namely, the one-sided controversy in criticism of the work of Sir Joseph Lister that was being carried on by Mr. Lawson Tait, the brilliant technician who was building a reputation by putting into practice the fundamental principles actually established by Lister. . . . I, a remote colonist of great England, realised that my remarks were not conventionally diplomatic but we all loved the mother country, and many of us overseas were astonished that so petty a quarrel could arise over so great a thing. We in America were cognizant of the value of Lawson Tait's work. . . . I asked the privilege of proposing the health of the other great surgeon who, though he was reluctant to give credit to the Master, nevertheless was instrumental in benefiting mankind by disseminating the principles of antiseptic and aseptic surgery, and I predicted that history

> would forget or forgive his criticism. There was profound silence, followed by many expressions of approval, punctuated with calls of "Hear! Hear!"
>
> In the midst of the confusion I finally succeeded in proposing the health of "one of England's most distinguished abdominal and pelvic surgeons – Mr. Lawson Tait, of Birmingham."
>
> It was difficult to determine whether or not I had made a faux pas, or if the preponderant partisanship caused them to forgive a foreigner his lack of diplomacy. At any rate they were polite and I received vigorous and rather long applause.

Martin states that Tait replied, but the incident is not recorded otherwise and it is perhaps unlikely that this attempt to honour Tait in his own country went down very well.

Tait did have many faithful adherents in Great Britain, but he seemed to be doomed to prominence as the leader of minorities, and when it came to matters such as seeking election to the Council of the College he was rejected. He could not, however, be ignored and his selection to give the address in Surgery to the British Medical Association when it met in Birmingham in 1890 was an indication of some appreciation of him and an honour which he himself considered as a recognition of his place in surgery. His speech, which was largely on surgical training, dwelt on the necessity of craftmanship. He talked at length about the skill of Birmingham artisans and suggested that any surgeon who hoped to develop real skill should emulate such workers and learn to use their tools. (Tait himself was skilled at the lathe and always had in his house a well equipped workshop.)

In 1890 he was awarded a joint prize by the two Royal Colleges in Edinburgh. This was a triennial award established by Dr. R.H. Gunning in the name of Cullen from the College of Physicians and in the name of Liston from the College of Surgeons. He received an elegant and valuable silver bowl with the citation "for the greatest benefit due to practical surgery in the triennial period".[2]

But Tait had made many enemies in high places. It served him ill that he had attacked , so vigorously and so vehemently, such respected leaders as Lister and Spencer Wells. His activities in the Medical Defence Union, the anti-vivisection movement and in so many other directions had not endeared him to many of his colleagues. In the atmosphere of jealousy and slander which still prevailed in the profession there were some individuals who were prepared to go to extremes to put him in his place. His downfall was primarily the result of three happenings. The first was a litigation brought against him by a Dr. Denholm, a general practitioner in Manchester. The second was the threat of an action concerning his alleged seduction of a nurse, with all the inevitable rumour and scandal. The third was a decline in the state of his health.

The Denholm v. Tait case was heard at the Manchester Assizes in 1892. Tait had been asked to see a patient previously under the care of this doctor who diagnosed a uterine tumour and treated it by electrolysis. The therapy was a failure and a serious complication developed. Tait advised operation and he removed the tumour. Forty-eight hours later the patient died unexpectedly. The husband tried to interview Tait but was handed a letter from him which read:[3]

> I saw your wife, with Mr. Christopher Martin, between two or three times this morning and matters were going on very fairly with her. At 7.30 I was summoned again and found her sinking. . . . The immediate cause of this unfortunate result is the rupture of a blood vessel at or near the spot where the electrical needles caused so much damaging inflammation or sloughing. Had she never been submitted to that treatment the case would have been a straightforward one and her recovery almost certain.

Not surprisingly, the husband attributed the death of his wife to improper treatment by Dr. Denholm before Tait's operation. For his part, Denholm regarded the letter as libellous. At the hearing evidence was given by the doctors who did the post mortem, that death was due to peritonitis. It was alleged, however, that the examination was inadequate, having been conducted by candlelight with the body remaining in a coffin! Tait stated that there had been a haemorrhage as a result of the operation and attributed this to the effects of Denholm's treatment. He denied that peritonitis had been proved as a complication, although he had not personally seen the autopsy. As a result of the evidence the plaintiff's case was withdrawn, but there were heavy costs charged to both sides.

Tait's letter to the patient's husband was hasty and ill-advised (although his counsel suggested it was honest and privileged and should not have been used against him). At that time he was fighting his battle against the use of electrical treatment for gynaecological conditions and his feelings were so strong that he may indeed have felt it his duty to expose Dr. Denholm. To many of his colleagues the letter to the patient's husband was seen as a libellous attack on a fellow practitioner. When it was learned that Tait's costs were being borne out of the scanty funds of the Medical Defence Union there was further criticism, especially because Tait had apparently agreed to refund such expenses. We have previously noted that the affair was followed by Tait's resignation of the presidency of the Union. Although technically he had been acquitted, his attitude throughout was viewed with considerable distrust. Those who were against him seized on the case with avidity (and probably not without pleasure), and even some of his friends wavered in their support.

While the Denholm case is well documented, much less is known of the more serious charge that he had assaulted one of his nurses. The full truth of this unsavoury episode remains uncertain. It is tempting to dismiss it as the type of slander which was all too common in the Victorian era. It is a curious coincidence that Sir James Simpson was involved in a similar situation, for he also was accused of fathering an illegitimate child. Although Simpson's case did not reach the law courts, the accusation was believed by many and was used against him by unscrupulous enemies. Inevitably this kind of rumour led to charges of habitual immorality against both Simpson and Tait.

The only printed evidence available to us concerning Tait's alleged misbehaviour is in a pamphlet which he sent to the Members of the Council of the British Medical Association early in 1895. He issued this to draw the attention of the Council to libellous statements made against him by Dr. Ernest Hart during a visit to the United States in 1893. Tait considered that Hart had gone to America in his official capacity of Editor of the *British Medical Journal,* and he demanded that the latter either prove that he did not make such statements or, if he admitted he had in fact done so, the Council should give Tait "consideration and protection." Tait had threatened Hart with a writ but withdrew it in the hope that the Association would deal with the matter.

In the preamble to the evidence produced in his pamphlet, Tait listed amongst many libels the charge of "suppressing deaths in the published records of my practice." In a series of letters reprinted in the pamphlet the more personal accusations appear. These letters followed an enquiry sent by Tait to Dr. Ernest Cushing, a Baltimore gynaecologist, in June 1894:[4]

Dear Sir,

At page 303, Vol. 130, of the Boston Medical and Surgical Journal you make the following reference to me "In the light of facts recently placed in evidence concerning Tait, his statistics have far less weight with the surgical world than was the case a year or two ago".

Would you be kind enough to inform me what these facts are, where they are placed in evidence, and the authority. . . .?

Dr. Cushing replied in September:

My information was received directly, and as a matter of fact of general knowledge, from a person very prominent in medical circles in England. . . . if what he said was true I submit that my expression was perfectly justifiable and my reference to the matter warranted, as it was not mentioned to me in confidence, nor under any reserve whatever. The alleged facts as related to me are briefly as follows:– that you were accused by a woman who had formerly been one of your nurses of having seduced her and of becoming the father of her illegitimate child. . . . that the case came into court and you evaded the support of the child under some legal defence, being compelled to admit, however, that it was your child; that these facts being "placed in evidence" you lost your professorship and your public hospital service and the most of your consultation practice. . . .

. . . .If I was deceived I owe you an apology and you may be assured that you will receive it and in as public a manner as that in which the aspersion on your reputation was given. . . . I will beg you to send me an account of the suit above referred to and the newspapers in which it was published, if it ever came into the newspapers.

On October 9th Tait replied in a remarkably fair manner:

I cannot but admire the frank and complete disclosure of your position nor can I refrain from sympathising with the unfortunate predicament in which you have been placed. But I cannot see, even if the story against me as you narrate it were true from beginning to end, what that can have to do with the trustworthiness of my statistics. . . .

As to the story: it is a lie, or rather a tissue of lies, from beginning to end. Two women, sisters, entered into a conspiracy to blackmail me; one [was] a nurse dismissed for insubordination and the other [was] one on whom I had done an ovariotomy, and they laid claim to £16,000 as hush money. They never got a stiver of that money for the reason you will see in the published account of it which I enclose. The case never came to trial, never a scrap of information appeared in the public press, much to my discomfort, but the plaintiffs' story was spread abroad as a means of coercing me to pay hush money, and chiefly by members of my own profession residing in London. . . . The plaintiffs traded on the belief that a man in my position and as rich as I was would pay up rather than have my name tarnished. But I would have spent my last shilling, and my wife would have sold her wedding ring, before I would have been bled in such a way. The case collapsed after nearly two years of legal dodging, and I never had the opportunity of proving the utter falseness of the charges made against me. Your informant may not have known this, but I expect he did. . .

. . . . I gave up my professorship because, as I said in my letter of resignation I did not ask for it – I did not want it – and I never valued it.

Finally I enclose a photographed copy of a complete withdrawal of the charges, signed by the woman who made them and witnessed by her attorney. . . .

You offer an apology and such reparation as is possible. I think as a man of honour you will do this and make as much reparation as lies in your power. But as a matter of right, I demand the name of my traducer, upon whom I shall inflict what correction his position may justify – that of friendly remonstrance in one case, that of vindictive prosecution in another.

Tait enclosed a copy of the letter of withdrawal of the charge from one Caroline Burnell. He enclosed also an extract of the annual report of 1893 of the Women's Hospital. In this report the resignation of Tait was accepted with great regret and with fulsome praise of his work in establishing the fame of the hospital. There was reference also to the exceptional results of abdominal operations with a mortality of 1.4 per cent in 142 recent cases. Perhaps Tait was rather naive in suggesting that if he was considered immoral in character this should not influence the reception of the published results of his operations. It was not, however, in the nature of his contemporaries either in Great Britain or America to accept the notion that a man could be honest in his professional claims and grossly immoral in his private life. Tait's reply was dignified and his protestations ring remarkably true.

There was one more enclosure with this letter of October 9th, 1894. This was an extract of an "Analysis of the Evidence in Seventy Cases of Charges made under the New Criminal Law Amendment Act: by Lawson Tait". This was published in the *Provincial Medical Journal* in 1894. The paper had been given to the Birmingham British Medical Association branch in October of the previous year. Tait had a grievance in that the laws of the country seemed to him to be biassed in favour of women so far as sexual offences were concerned. To illustrate the frequency of blackmail in relation to charges of sexual crime he recounted what seems quite clearly to have been his own experience. It was rather curious that he did this, for his Birmingham audience must have been aware of the charge against him. Was this public statement made out of sheer bravado or was it made to emphasise his innocence? The extract reads:[5]

> An English surgeon had occasion some seven years ago to take a continental journey for the purpose of performing a special operation, and he took with him a nurse who had been years in his service. . . . Five years after she had been dismissed from his service, she and her sister conspired to extort a large sum of money, £8,000, as blackmail, on a charge that on the journey in question he filled her with wine and took undue advantage of her: that she bore a child, which was his. His instructions were at once to institute criminal proceedings for conspiracy to extort, but every lawyer consulted by him advised strongly against this course. . . . To none of these advisers would he listen, and a writ containing the infamous charges was issued, and copies of it and other documents were freely exhibited, in the hope that the half public scandal would prove to be sufficiently coercive. At last he obtained the proof that they had not travelled together, but the time had elapsed in which criminal proceedings could be taken and nothing remained but an action for perjury if the plaintiff persisted in the story of the writ. This brought the parties involved to a proper state of mind, and the result was a letter of complete and unconditional withdrawal of all imputations against the persistent defendant.

This extract places the alleged incident about 1887 and it seems likely that rumours of an impending action were spread around from 1890 onwards.

Dr. Cushing replied promptly to Tait's letter of explanation:

> . . . to say that I was surprised at the contents of the letter and the enclosure is putting it very mildly. . . . it is clear that my informant has lied to me most damnably and maliciously about you, and that you can settle with him. But he has moreover made a fool of me and led me into a false position and that he has to settle with me. . . .

> He also told me that your statements were not credited in regard to your results by the best part of the profession in England, that you had lost all your practice and taken to heavy drinking, and more things to the discredit of your reputation.
>
> .... My informant then was Dr. Ernest Hart, Editor of the British Medical Journal, and great instructor of the American profession in all matters of medical ethics and proprieties. He told me of the above alleged facts and various other things to your discredit when we were travelling together in the excursion of the Pan-American Medical Congress from Washington to Chicago, a little over a year ago. There was no reserve or request that the facts should not be repeated. I had every reason to believe that Dr. Hart knew what he was talking about and it never entered my mind that he was not telling the truth....

Dr. Cushing admitted that Hart's information had caused him to doubt Tait's surgical records, but he offered a full apology and said that he would give any evidence necessary if an action was taken against Hart. To this letter Tait replied on November 8th, 1894:

> ....I must express some reserve as to the unquestioned acceptance you seem to have given to Mr. Ernest Hart's statements .... it would be a surprise to me if you were not aware of the fiery discussions that have taken place in this country on the question of vivisection, in which Mr. Ernest Hart and I have taken entirely opposite views. A more domestic incident, but one quite as much to the purpose is the recent trouble in the Medical Defence Union, a matter which, though it is not likely to be familiar to you, is none the less calculated to suggest that any statement of Mr. Ernest Hart having reference to me or my work must necessarily be received with caution.

Tait went on to suggest that since Hart, as Editor of the *Journal*, had published many of his papers he had no right now to suggest that the statistics were unreliable. He asked Dr. Cushing to publicise a full retraction in the *Boston Medical Journal*. No such apology seems to have appeared.

Tait's appeal, with the pamphlet, went before the Journal and Finance Committee of the Association in January 1895. A letter was read from the solicitor who acted for the Association:[6]

> In my opinion, as I have already stated, the matter is not an Association matter but a personal one between Mr. Lawson Tait and Mr. Ernest Hart and is not, therefore, one which the Council is under any obligation to discuss.
>
> I may cite in support of this opinion that Mr. Lawson Tait issued his writ against Mr. Hart and not against the Association and that Mr. Hart placed himself in the hands of his private solicitors and did not directly or indirectly consult myself.

The committee moved that Lawson Tait's complaints against Hart were matters outside the jurisdiction of the Association and the Council adopted this recommendation on the same day. Very probably the Council was greatly relieved that it could wriggle out of the situation on this legal advice. The decision must have disappointed Tait, but he accepted it without public complaint and he did not resign from the Association as might have been expected. From this time onwards Tait does not appear to have taken any further positive action to clear his name.

Dr. Hart must clearly be criticised adversely for libelling Tait in this way, particularly as he most likely knew that there was a threat of legal action and that the case was therefore *sub judice.* Hart, although he had accepted so many of Tait's papers, had given him a bad press on matters concerning vivisection and the Medical Defence Union. It was Tait's weakness that he should so readily enter into a personal vendetta with anyone like Hart, who disagreed with him on professional matters.

Ernest Hart (1835-1898) was an unusual man. Of Jewish parentage, he had qualified at St. George's Hospital and practised as a surgeon for some years. He was attracted to medical journalism and served on the staff of the *Lancet* until 1866, when he transferred his allegiance to the *British Medical Journal,* of which he at once became Editor. Through the columns of the *Journal* he advocated reforms of all kinds with a fervency which rivalled that of Thomas Wakley of the *Lancet* in earlier years. He spared no one in furthering his causes. He was described as possessing "an incisive eloquence which was the admiration of his friends and the dread of his enemies—for a man of his calibre was sure to have enemies." There was a scandal in 1868 when he was charged with appropriating certain funds of the Association. He resigned as Editor of the *Journal,* but was reinstated by the Council a year later without explanation and without any questions being asked. Under his management the *Journal* prospered and a large increase in membership of the Association was attributed to him.

Hart has been described variously as rash, self-assured, freebooting and raffish. He was unpopular with many members of the profession, scandal was spread about his activities and religious prejudice was exerted against him. There were some strange rumours concerning the death of his first wife in 1857, after only two years of marriage. He was nevertheless a very powerful influence in medical affairs. The last years of his life were spent in chronic invalidism: he suffered from diabetes, then an uncontrollable disease. This may have accounted for unstable or ill-judged actions on his part.[7]

The details of this regrettable episode are given in full because it seems certain that it had more to do with Tait's downfall than had any other factor. Happening when Tait was already exposed to censure over the Denholm case, it inevitably had serious repercussions. Rumour is a much more sinister influence in such situations than is an event which comes into full publicity. In the many modern biographies of eminent Victorians, few seem to escape the charges of immoral or perverted sexual behaviour. Not infrequently such allegations came to light in their lifetime—for example, in the case of Sir Charles Dilke the politician. The extent to which professional or other well-known men indulged in unlicensed or immoral activities in this age is uncertain. The veneer of respectability and moral rectitude seems to have been fragile. The background of vice and crime of the underworld of the large cities and the considerable involvement in this of men from the upper social strata cannot be denied. Of this period it has been suggested that "the specifically sexual inhibitions of ordinary society, its general prudishness and formality produced their own counter effects."[8] In such a background the weapon of blackmail was frequently exploited. It is possible that Tait was the victim of just such an unjustified attack of this kind by a nurse who in some way offended him and who had been peremptorily dismissed from his service. Whether innocent or guilty, it was certain that malicious rumours concerning Tait's morals would spread, and it is also certain that as a result he could never again be completely reinstated socially or professionally.[9]

Contemporary opinion of Tait's morality (or immorality) may have had some basis in fact, but such adverse reports as exist could well be groundless, having been stimulated by the rumour of this one alleged act of moral delinquency.

Of his friends and admirers, Christopher Martin had a good opinion of Tait: "He enjoyed the good things of life; but he was neither a gourmand nor a drunkard. . . . He was as clean in his mind as in his person: I never saw him reading an immoral book, nor heard him tell a dirty story". In his biography of Tait, McKay makes no direct allusion to the scandal which influenced his life so greatly. In his uncompleted autobiography, however, McKay describes how a lady in Ireland, having read in the biography about a peculiarity of Tait's fingers, wrote to McKay insisting that she was Tait's illegitimate daughter. As evidence she sent an outline of her fingers which were exactly the shape of those of Tait! McKay advised her to write to Christopher Martin and alleges that "he sent her the absolute proof she required."

Francis Brett Young, in his novel, drops strong hints of profligacy and lewdness in Tait's character; however, these may be entirely fictional. Professor Leonard Gamgee (1868-1956) of Birmingham, who was well informed about Tait, discussed him with his grandson, who recalls, "I can well see him now after five minutes of discussion of Lawson Tait and the abdomen suddenly say 'but there were other things', then a knowing shake of his head, 'his Private affairs I mean'".[10] These are only hints and could be based on mere rumour. Rumour, however, was powerful and left a tarnished image of Tait which has never been removed.

Tait's real affection for his wife is brought out in many accounts. She in her turn may have overcome any suspicion or knowledge of infidelity by intense loyalty or generous forgiveness. She was childless, which could tempt one to suggest that Tait's reaction to this sad fact may have led him to relax his principles. After so many years the truth eludes us and we cannot sit in judgement on the basis of the evidence available to us. Of one thing we may be certain: Tait, before he was fifty years of age, had lost his influence, his practice and much of his zest for life. Christopher Martin, who may well have known all the facts, sums up the situation: "Whether this story was true or false there can be no doubt it did him a tremendous amount of harm".

Tait's medical history at this time is significant. A comparison of his portraits before and after 1890 reveal a change from a powerful and virile individual to one of a rather corpulent and flabby appearance. When Tait wrote to Cushing in October 1894 he stated: "During the weary progress of the case I became the victim of a stone in the kidney and I was laid off work for six months, and this gave colour to the story of my leaving my practice". Certainly in 1892 his appearances in London at meetings of organisations such as the British Gynaecological Society were very infrequent. In the same year he went for a while to Hampshire to convalesce and then travelled to Italy for his health.

McKay suggests that Tait began to have trouble from stones in the kidney about 1890 and that it was this which induced him to slow the pace of his activities. Gilbert Barling (1855-1940), surgeon to the Birmingham Hospital, operated to remove a urethral stone in 1897. Christopher Martin records some details which suggest that Tait was a rather difficult patient:[11]

> Mr. Tait took the anaesthetic badly, went black in the face and nearly died. Immediately after the operation Mr. Barling went on holiday and left him in my charge. Needless to say I told him to keep to a bland milky diet and stay absolutely in bed. Next day, however, a friend (Dr. Donovan) called and found him sitting by the fire in a dressing-gown, with a Tam-o-Shanter on his head, a big cigar in his mouth, and a pint of champagne at his elbow. "Hello", said Donovan, "is this allowed?" "Oh, yes", said Tait, "Christopher ordered it". In spite of this and his refusal to allow me to use antiseptics, he made a good recovery. On the fifth day he got up and, though it was bitterly cold weather, insisted in driving out to his bungalow at Yardley Wood – against Mrs. Tait's entreaties and my protests. After his arrival he sent me this defiant telegram, "Arrived safely, temperature normal, had beef and pickles for dinner".

There was an illness about 1891 when Tait developed a septic hand from an operation wound with severe inflammation of the axillary glands and septicaemia. He thought at one stage that he might not recover. Gilbert Barling, in reminiscences of Tait's life, describes how he saw him at this time and also records that there was "a very suspicious sore" on his hand.[12] There is considerable evidence that Tait developed chronic nephritis after this illness, which could well have been the sequel to an acute nephritis from septicaemia. Tait's appearance after 1890 certainly suggests this diagnosis. There is no evidence that Tait became an alcoholic, as was suggested to Cushing by Hart.

In 1893 Tait resigned his post as surgeon to the Women's Hospital, but he was retained as a consultant surgeon. Shortly after he gave up his professorship. He relinquished his presidency of the Birmingham Medical Institute and of the Medical Defence Union. His private practice declined rapidly, partly due to his periods of illness but mainly, it would seem, because of defamatory statements concerning his character. He found himself in financial difficulty and had to sell his house in the New Forest, his yacht on the Solent and his collection of antiques. For a while he continued to practise from the Crescent, but he had to cut down the staff of his private hospital to about a third. It may be that he had lived in such style that he had squandered all his large income and had saved none of it. Certainly his lavish establishments must have cost him a great deal of money. It is possible that he was affected by a financial crisis which hit the country in 1892, but we have no hint of his dabbling in the stock markets. The possibility cannot be dismissed that he did pay hush money to his accusers and that this exhausted such reserves as were available to him. In addition, he undoubtedly incurred heavy costs over his various legal actions.

Between 1892 and 1895 Tait's appearances at the medical societies were intermittent and his flow of letters and articles lessened. There were a few notes on individual cases, but such articles as he wrote offered nothing original or of great importance. There were still sporadic outbursts attacking Listerism, the conservative school of surgery and those who used animal experiments in their research. He continued also to be involved in personal quarrels which he conducted in the correspondence columns of the medical press. Spencer Wells died in 1897; Tait often expressed regret that he and Wells had quarrelled, but he never forgave Wells for his terse criticism of his (Tait's) advocacy of surgical removal of the diseased appendages. The two men had moved in different worlds. Wells was widely accepted in society; he was also a Baronet, surgeon to the Queen's Household, President of the Royal College of Surgeons, Elder Statesman of British Surgery and the acknowledged leader of the medical profession in London. Tait, on the other hand, was the provincial surgeon–to some a brash opportunist and social climber–leader of minority oppositions to established institutions and ideas and never fully accepted for his influence on surgery.

Around 1891 Gladstone offered Tait a baronetcy, probably in some recognition of his political activities, but Tait refused. A report in a Wakefield paper reads:

> It is stated on unquestionable authority, that Mr. Lawson Tait of Birmingham, who is well known and much respected in this neighbourhood (having family relationships with Wakefield) was recently offered a baronetcy in recognition of his distinguished services to surgical science. The honour however has been respectfully declined. A contemporary comments as follows:— "The offer does equal honour both to the Prime Minister and to Mr. Tait. In his department of surgery Mr. Lawson Tait ranks with the highest, and such a recognition of his brilliant services to obstetric science would, we

> think, have been appreciated by his professional brethren. Mr. Tait is however a man of strong individuality, and rather prides himself on his eclecticism in most matters. He is fond of associating himself with the minority on almost any question, a preference which probably accounts for the fact that in Unionist Birmingham he elects to be a Gladstonian. But he enjoys respect for the candour and independence of his character. He owes much of his professional success to his daring originality, and he differs from most Radicals, in setting a light value upon titular distinction".

It seems likely that Tait did consider accepting the honour, for about 1890 a commemorative copper medal was struck with an excellent likeness of Tait on the obverse and on the reverse a prospective and appropriate coat of arms including formalised surgical knots. It was designed by the Birmingham medallist Joseph Moore (1817-1882), who was a close friend of Tait and who had a considerable reputation in England for this type of work.

Tait's life had changed from the hectic round of hospital practice and private work to consultations all over the country, which he himself had described: "I move about the country to an extent that almost equals the work of a commercial traveller". Much of his fire had gone, for he was a tired man, and before he reached the age of fifty he was prematurely old. His private hospital at the Crescent was gradually closed down, but he retained to the end of his days a consulting room in Newhall Street in Birmingham. He left the Crescent and lived in a small house in Yardley Wood in the suburbs until 1897. He did continue to make some sort of a living, for many practitioners in Birmingham – and even in London – remained faithful and called him for consultation. He went on operating on private patients, but he was no longer performing the huge annual totals of abdominal procedures with which he had astonished the world. He was never to regain his former position in the surgical world.

CHAPTER X

Last Years

When some of the dust had settled after the unhappy disturbances of the previous years it seemed around 1896 that Tait's fortunes might revive. He announced that he was once more working at the second volume of his text on abdominal surgery. He was also seeking material for a biography of the ovariotomist Charles Clay, for he wanted to accord to Clay belated credit for his pioneer work. However, neither project was completed. Meanwhile the flow of letters to the medical press continued. Most of these were written to criticise other gynaecologists, usually with a strong indication that Tait had settled the particular issue already. His readers were constantly reminded of his past achievements, and he seemed determined that he would not be forgotten. There were many more letters on medico-political, medico-legal and other general topics. The General Medical Council was attacked over its attitude to unqualified assistants. Animal experimentation was still condemned with special reference to current investigations on the effects of chloroform. Of these he wrote, "I beg that the columns of our journal be no more wasted in this endless wrangle about the action of various anaesthetics on animals. They differ *toto coelo* in their actions respectively in different animals: and those actions are in no way comparable to the results seen in mankind". He entered into discussion on the liquor laws, his intervention being duly noted in a leader in the *Lancet* with the comment that the controversy was "enlivened by the evidence of Mr. Lawson Tait who may generally be relied on to strike out a line of his own."[1] Despite his semi-retirement his opinions were still to be heard. He advanced very sound views about the problem of alcoholism in women and produced statistics proving that female inebriation was most frequent at or near the age of fifty. He condemned treatment by sudden deprivation of alcohol and deplored the fact that women under a new Government Bill might be put in prison because they were alcoholics. He believed that many such unfortunates owed their condition to untreated or badly treated pelvic disease, and he seized the opportunity once more of attacking conservative or medical treatment of such chronic inflammations, pressing his views on radical operation. As always, he showed his compassion towards his patients, especially those whose lives were made unbearable by a failure to diagnose and eradicate the cause of mental or physical deterioration.

In the last four years of his life Tait seldom reported clinical cases to the London Societies, but he did continue to contribute at meetings of the Birmingham Medical Institute. It may be surmised that he was still accepted as a stimulating member of this local group of doctors, many of whom still felt respect and consideration for him.

Tait's inventive genius had not deserted him. Compared with many of his contemporaries he was not prone to excessive modifications of existing instruments or apparatus but always prided himself on the simplicity of his surgical equipment. A list of the instruments he evolved is short, and most were of real practical value. He had devised an apparatus for the administration of ether, but since the ether was vaporised by an open spirit lamp this must have been rather a dangerous piece of equipment! He produced his own modification of artery forceps, special wire snares or ligatures for the more difficult vascular pedicles, a corkscrew to assist in the removal of solid uterine tumors, drainage tubes, and a special cannula for evacuating the contents of cysts. In 1896 he devised an "electric haemostat" for controlling bleeding, an advance on Keith's method of cauterising the pedicle by heat. There was an ingenious "vaginal stethoscope" by which he alleged he could detect "faint pelvic sounds" to diagnose early pregnancy. His final offering was the "Lawson Tait Bedstead", used for many years in most hospitals and the subject of his last paper.

In his many letters Tait reiterated his firm views on certain priorities in surgical history. He was determined to credit Houston of Glasgow with the first successful ovariotomy—erroneously, as we have suggested. He insisted that his former chief Mackenzie Edwards should be given the priority for devising the muscle-splitting technique for exposure of the kidney, a priority usually awarded to Mayo Robson. To Edwards he awarded also the credit for establishing the use of lumbar colostomy in Great Britain.

In 1896 Tait published a long paper in which he made a vigorous attempt to put surgical history straight. In this survey, entitled "The Evolution of the Surgical Treatment of the Broad Ligament Pedicle", he remarks that the whole story of abdominal surgery, "in the slow tardy evolution of its first stages, turned on the treatment of the broad ligament pedicle." He reminds his readers that the American surgeon Nathan Smith, when removing an ovarian cyst (in 1822), cut the ligatures short but that no one appreciated this advance. Once more he condemns Spencer Wells for his long advocacy of the use of the external crushing clamp. To himself and Bantock, Tait gives the credit for the final establishment of the use of the short ligature with the vascular pedicle returned to the abdomen.

Few of Tait's last papers appeared in the *British Medical Journal* or the *Lancet*, but for such rather discursive reviews he found a new medium in the popular but less authoritative *Medical Press and Circular.* To this he contributed a paper entitled "The Evolution of the Aseptic Method of Surgery". This was his last round in the quarrel with Lister, and it claimed that Tait was largely responsible for the introduction of the concept of aseptic surgery which, in his opinion, owed little to Lister and much to Syme and Simpson.

By now there were fewer invitations to lecture throughout the country, but it must have given Tait great pleasure to return to Wakefield. There, in 1897, he gave a paper on myomatous tumours of the uterus to the local medical society and indulged in some reminiscences of his surgical apprenticeship in the Wakefield Hospital.

The year 1897 marked the Diamond Jubilee of Victoria's reign. It was the occasion for elaborate reviews of developments in all the Arts and Sciences. In Medicine there had been unprecedented advances and there was justifiable pride in the achievements of the glorious sixty years. The *British Medical Journal* had a commemoration number in June with full accounts of the progress of Medical Science. In the section on surgery the writer saw the period as a Golden Age with Paget's contributions to surgical pathology, Lister's introduction of antiseptic surgery and the discovery of general anaesthesia as the most significant events.[2] The rise of abdominal surgery was also acclaimed as an important development and Tait was linked with Frederic Treves, Mayo Robson and Knowsley Thornton as having expanded the pioneer work of the ovariotomists such as Charles Clay and Spencer Wells. While some mention was made of the importance of the practice of discarding the long ligature in ovariotomy, Tait's part in this was not recognised. In the sections on obstetrics and gynaecology the main credit for advances in abdominal procedures was accorded to Spencer Wells. Although Tait was recognised for his introduction of the radical operation for removal of diseased appendages, the reference was rather oblique: "Lawson Tait overstepped the limits of ovarian tumours". There was a strong hint that his teaching had resulted in wholesale and unjustified removal of the ovaries. In a paragraph on ectopic pregnancy there was, rather unjustly, no mention of his dramatic success in the management of the acute case.

The *Lancet* had a less detailed survey.[3] In the surgical section Tait's name was linked with that of Marion Sims as a pioneer in the surgery of the gallbladder, but Tait was not mentioned in the section on gynaecology.

Contemporaries in 1897 clearly did not accord much credit to Tait for his part in the evolution of surgery or gynaecology. In the final chapter (immediately following) we shall consider whether or not the contributors to these special issues of the journals were fair in their assessment.

In 1897 there was a change in Tait's domestic life. He purchased some land near Llandudno and built to his own design a house, St. Petrock's.[4] It still stands on the cliff side of the Great Orme with a magnificent view of the mountains and the sea. The site had prehistoric associations which must have appealed to him, with an ancient monument known as Gogarth's cave. He had already given up his consulting room and his private hospital at the Crescent and had sold his house in Yardley Wood. He travelled twice or thrice a week from Llandudno to Birmingham to consult at his rooms in Newall Street or to attend the Institute meetings. His journeys South were now few, but he still retained his hospital consultancy in Southampton. He continued to operate, occasionally in London, but usually in or near Birmingham. In 1898 he reported with some pride that he had performed yet another Porro procedure, and that both mother and child had survived. It must be presumed that these operations were done in small private nursing homes since he no longer had access to public or private beds of his own.

He still had plans for the future, including the establishment of a sanatorium near Llandudno for tubercular patients. He entered into local affairs with his usual gusto and was active as a member of an association to improve the tourist attractions of Llandudno.[5] Despite his indifferent health he seemed to have established a new life and accepted his limitations.

Tait's last paper, published in the *Birmingham Medical Review* of 1899, was a long and entertaining study entitled "The Bedstead as an important factor in domestic hygiene and comfort". He traced the history of the bed from the cave-dweller to modern times. He attributed much of the pestilence (particularly typhus) of early centuries to the unsanitary overcrowding of wooden four-poster beds, which were enclosed in suffocating hanging curtains. He applauded the introduction of single beds, which he attributed to the French around 1850. He had very firm opinions about the desirability of metal bedsteads and of adequate ventilation in the bedroom. He had introduced the "Lawson Tait" bedstead, designed so that it was a convenient height from the floor. It had a firm wire mattress which did not sag, and could be easily moved about in house or hospital on footpads of india rubber rather than on castors, which were not only noisy but frequently came off. Tait's became the standard bed in hospitals for many years.

In Birmingham, on May 26 1899, Tait performed what proved to be his last operation. He went to Droitwich on June 3rd on the occasion of the opening of a new railway station. A guest at the lunch which followed, Tait spoke briefly: "I came to Droitwich last night: I was quite well, I had a bath and today I am better".

The end came suddenly; just ten days later (June 13th) while at Llandudno, Tait was seized with severe pain following a brief illness. There were rumours that two eminent London specialists were summoned, but in fact Tait remained under the care of a local practitioner. Although he was uraemic he retained full consciousness and no doubt told his doctor exactly what he thought about his own case. He knew he was dying and faced his end coolly and courageously. He took his last cigar with the announcement that "I am smoking a very good Larranaga—and the last I shall ever smoke". He expired quite suddenly that same afternoon.

His death was certified as due to chronic nephritis and uraemia. It seems likely that there was a calculus obstruction with complete suppression of his already deficient renal function. The final illness bears out the diagnoses made a few years previously.

Tait apparently left careful instructions about his funeral arrangements, which gave rise to some publicity and confusion. He had directed that his body be buried in Gogarth's cave behind his house. The local authorities objected, so the family appealed to the Home Secretary. A compromise was reached, both parties agreeing that his remains be cremated and the ashes deposited in the cave. Accordingly, his body was taken to Liverpool accompanied by only three mourners—his brother-in-law Martin Stewart, and two legal gentlemen. Tait had directed that there be no mourning coaches, no funeral attire and no religious service. His cremation was the sixth performed at the newly built crematorium at Anfield.[7] The urn containing the ashes was brought to Llandudno. Five years later Mrs. Tait arranged for a reburial of the ashes in Warriston Cemetery in Edinburgh, but there is a record of a memorial tablet placed at the entrance to the cave, bearing the inscription:

The Grave of Lawson Tait.

In this cave reposes the urn containing the ashes of Lawson Tait, after cremation. It was his wish that he should be buried in this romantic spot, within the grounds surrounding his new home at Llandudno, North Wales

The local papers recorded his funeral in some detail, perhaps a little disapproving of its austerity. The argument about the disposal of the ashes created considerable speculation. The *Llandudno Courier* sent a reporter to interview Mrs. Tait; he found that she was "bearing up well" although she was somewhat resentful that it had been reported that no flowers should be sent, for she said her husband had loved flowers. Mrs. Tait refused to divulge what had been done with the urn.

The final resting place of Tait's ashes in Warriston Cemetery is marked by a Celtic Cross with the simple inscription:

In Memoriam
Lawson Tait, F.R.C.S.
Born in Edinburgh May 1845
Died at St. Petrock's, Llandudno, 13th June 1899

Mrs. Tait died in 1909 at Exmouth and was buried in the same grave. Her name and the details of her birth were added to the tombstone with the somewhat cryptic tribute "She hath done what she could". The grave is very near that of Sir James Young Simpson. Although Tait had finally directed that his remains be placed in Gogarth's cave, his widow perhaps carried out an earlier wish. This detail of the interment of his ashes near the Simpson grave revives the enigma concerning Tait's parentage.

He had made a will in 1893 leaving everything to his wife. The gross value was only £9,571, a meagre total for a consultant surgeon of his time.[9]

The suddenness of Lawson Tait's death took the medical world by surprise. Although he was known to suffer chronic ill health, he was only 54 years of age. There were full obituaries in both the lay and the medical press. In our final chapter it remains to comment on contemporary opinions of Tait at his death and to offer a new evaluation of his character and achievement some 75 years later.

CHAPTER XI

Achievement and Character: A Retrospective Assessment

Some assessment has already been made of the acceptance or rejection of Lawson Tait by the profession in his lifetime. Contemporary opinion can be measured also from the obituaries, although these may be biassed according to the personal views of the writer. Soon after death, interest in the career of a notable person is often lost although, for some, criticism or even denigration may be accentuated. A generation later there is a revival of interest and often a reinstatement in terms of importance or influence. As far as technical achievements are concerned we can in retrospect readily measure the influence of a surgeon on the progress of his specialty.

Obituaries in the lay press have a news value and current events may influence the space given to them or the interest engendered by them. When Lawson Tait died two major topics dominated the newspapers. One was the reprieve of the French Army officer Alfred Dreyfus, whose case had been followed with great interest in England. The other was the celebration of the eightieth birthday of Queen Victoria. An almost mystical attitude had developed towards the Queen, which was accentuated by the likelihood of her survival into a new century. On June 14th the *Times* printed a rather meagre notice of Tait's death. It was conceded that "he brought into existence a large number of new operations for diseases of the abdomen and perfected many others." No details of his work were given, nor was there any hint that a unique personality had passed from the scene. The news value of his death was enhanced by the dilemma concerning the disposal of his remains, and indeed two days later there was a quite a long paragraph about this matter.

If the *Times* failed to give Tait much notice, the Birmingham papers were more generous. The *Birmingham Daily Gazette* devoted several columns to "Birmingham's distinguished surgeon and citizen."[1] His career was traced with reasonable accuracy and his contributions to surgery were enumerated and fairly assessed. There were also many reminiscences and anecdotes which emphasised his unusual character. The *Birmingham Post* was equally laudatory concerning Tait's achievements and added its quota of anecdotes.[2] Birmingham certainly appreciated the fact that her best known and most public-spirited citizen had died and that the world had lost a great surgeon.

The Liverpool papers reported in full the drama of Tait's death for the particular benefit of their readers in North Wales. A special tribute from "an Old Pupil" suggested that "the surgical profession had lost its ablest son."[3] There was a reference to Tait's battle with the London surgeons: "to see him turn up at a crack London Scientific Society attired in a snuff-coloured coat, tartan necktie and variegated combinations [sic] was a sight for the gods and this flouting was deliberately done". The anonymous contributor, perhaps Dr. Hawkins-Ambler, who had settled as a gynaecologist in Liverpool after being with Tait in Birmingham, recalled the struggle against vivisection and how Tait had hoped that on his tombstone would be inscribed that "he laboured to divert his profession from the blundering of experiments in the sub-human groups of animal life in the hope that they would shed light on the aberrant physiology of the human group."

A popular Penny Weekly, *M.A.P.* ("Mainly About People"), edited by the journalist T. P. O'Connor, printed a few paragraphs about Tait. He was described as "a strange, picturesque creature, with many ardent enemies, and with many warm friends." His almost manic activity was emphasised: "it was a life of mad energy, of deadly and destructive work, that in the end brought down the magnificent and Titanic frame and put him in a premature grave". O'Connor could not resist some speculation on the topic of Tait's origins:[4]

> One of the stories about him was that he was the natural son of the late Sir James Simpson .... Lawson Tait used to speak of the report himself—he was not a reticent creature—but at the same time laughingly would contradict it. And yet there was never a likeness so pronounced as between these two men.... I saw Simpson once ... and I can still remember the man, though it is thirty years ago, with his large face, his great bull head, his shaggy looks, his short stout body, in other words, I can see him the very image of Lawson Tait.

O'Connor may have known Tait well but he offered no real proof to support the story of illegitimacy. Like McKay, he made a lot of a resemblance to Tait in the figure portrayed by the statue of Simpson which stands at the West End of Princes Street in Edinburgh. This was scarcely a convincing piece of evidence. This journalistic gossip drew a reply from "a member of the family of the late Sir James Simpson." This may have been written by his nephew Sir Alexander Simpson or by his daughter Eve:[5]

> I write on behalf of the surviving members of the family of the late Sir James Simpson in regard to the statement contained in your issue of the 24th June to the effect that one of the stories about the late Mr. Lawson Tait was "that he was a natural son of Sir James Simpson, the great Scotch physician". There is not the slightest foundation for this story. Sir James Simpson was a man of irreproachable character, and the statement made by you is calculated to bring dishonour on his memory, as it has given pain to his surviving relatives. Mr. Tait was a favourite student of Sir James Simpson. They were men of kindred genius, but this was the only kinship. The genuine parentage of Mr. Tait is recorded in the books of Heriot's Hospital, where he was brought up, and there is no ground for the rumour that he was illegitimate.

We turn now to the obituaries in the medical press. The *British Medical Journal*, in a preliminary notice, referred to Tait with some generosity: "He has written his name large on the history of the great development of surgery which has taken place during the last quarter of a century".[6] In the longer notice which followed there were acknowledgements of his achievements in surgery and gynaecology, but hints of difficulties arising from his personality: "He showed a want of respect for age and authority, remarkable even for Birmingham". Of his eclipse in 1892 it was written, somewhat evasively:[7]

> The financial crisis of 1892 apparently affected him seriously, for in the immediate succeeding years all sorts of rumours appeared about him in the press. No great surgical position was ever lost more rapidly or lost with such pathetic suddenness. He was to leave Birmingham and settle in London or America, and all sorts of other stories floated about.

The *Lancet* recorded with some eloquence that "the unexpected death of Mr. Lawson Tait. . . . has removed from the domain of surgery a light which has shone with singular force and brilliancy for a number of years." He was given due credit for his surgical dexterity and his originality. The surgical address to the British Medical Association in 1890 was recalled: "in it we see his clear-headedness, his pugnacity, his contempt for detail, his worship of good surgery and his glory in his own talents". Of his pugnacity we read: "He dearly loved a losing cause and a concensus [sic] of opinion was anathema to him".[8]

The *Medical Press* wrote: "Great Britain has been deprived of the most original surgeon she has produced in the last quarter of a century and the whole world of surgery has to deplore the loss of one of the most gifted masters of the art". There was a generous recognition of his talents and his achievements, with an oblique *caveat*: "we have naught to say to certain personal attributes which brought him many and relentless enemies. His best friends . . . . would have often wished that in debate and in medical literature his attitude in scientific discussion were other than it was".[9]

The President of the Obstetrical Society of London, Alban Doran (1849-1927), in his annual address to the Society, gave a very full account of Tait's early life and training (perpetuating the erroneous suggestion that Tait's father was a lawyer and a cousin of the Archbishop of Canterbury). Doran appreciated Tait's success and originality in dealing with chronically inflamed tubes and ovaries by radical surgery. He measured Tait's contribution to the surgery of ruptured ectopic pregnancy generously: "Nobody can deny that Tait conferred on womenkind great benefit by his boldness in the treatment of ectopic gestation: this truth is proved by the wonderful advance in the surgery of this condition during the past seventeen years". In this and in many other things Tait's influence was recognised fully, but then came the cautionary remarks: "his influence in the profession was by no means in all respects satisfactory. He was no man of science like Huxley, the pure scientist, or Paget, the surgeon who knew how to apply science to surgery . . . . Tait was too eager to make scientific facts appear to support his personal views and justify his practices". There were other criticisms. He was accused of operating unnecessarily in many cases and of using inaccurate statistical methods. "His manner of conducting disputes was, to say the least, unconcilitary [sic] . . . . Yet Lawson Tait did great things and will not be forgotten".[10]

Most accounts made no reference to the disasters in Tait's life, but the *Practitioner* was the exception. In a short editorial Tait's death was commented upon somewhat unsympathetically:[11]

> Another surgical writer who was always readable, however much one might differ from the opinions and sentiments he expressed, has passed away in poor Lawson Tait. Nature had been prodigal of intel-

> lectual gifts; and assuredly he did not hide his light under a bushel. Yet his last years were spent in a fruitless struggle to regain a lost position . . . . his professional sun had sunk below the horizon. What this occultation was due to is a subject which I do not feel called upon to discuss, nor is it for me to enforce the moral of his career.

Such was the style of the tributes which appeared in 1899. While in most there was an opening statement granting Tait a place in surgical history, the acknowledgement was often given grudgingly and was always followed by reservations. This is understandable; Tait in 1899 was to some extent already a forgotten man; he had not died at the height of his powers, as might have been expected in a man of 54. Much had happened since he had introduced his original ideas, and it was still too early to assess his influence on the rapid changes in all branches of surgery. His flouting of convention as well as his attacks on established institutions had not been forgotten (nor entirely forgiven). His support of Darwinism in earlier years, his opposition to Lister, his part in the antivivisection movement and so many other things had left a legacy of disapproval. Not least, the allegations against his morals—and even his pleasure in associating with the theatrical world—accentuated criticism and suspicion. Few of his contemporaries were prepared to be more than lukewarm about his achievements, for they could not divorce his eccentricities and his private life from his professional activities. The further from London, however, the more generous were the tributes.

On September 20th (1899) Charles Reed delivered "A Memorial Address on the Life and Character of Lawson Tait" to the American Association of Obstetricians and Gynaecologists. Tait had been made a Fellow of this association and the tribute was an index of American regard for him. Reed recalled how he first learned of Tait through his book on the diseases of women, which reached America in 1877. He described how the orthodox gynaecology which he had been taught and which he then practised was futile, but that "the first light came to him in the little book from Birmingham – and the darkness began to dissipate." The American gynaecologist had visited Tait in 1886 to see his methods at first hand. He spent some weeks in Birmingham "replete with valuable experience, delightful personal association and cordial hospitality, so that when my leave-taking came I felt I was leaving the home 'neath whose roof I had imbibed the inspiration for my life work." He summed up Tait's life and work:[12]

> It may be said of Mr. Tait that he laid the foundation of modern abdominal and pelvic surgery: that he personally devised the chief operations that pertain to that department of practice: that he invented many new instruments and improved many others: that he refined surgical technique to its present simplicity; that he demonstrated for the first time much of the now accepted pathology of the uterine appendages; that he reduced the mortality in abdominal and pelvic surgery to the minimum; that he, more than any other one man forced the reforms whereby modern hospitals have been brought to their present high state of efficiency and finally, that he has added many years of life and happiness not only to women, but to mankind.

This was a much more generous tribute than any accorded in Great Britain. It certainly reflected the opinion of the many American surgeons who came under Tait's influence directly (by visiting him in Birmingham) or indirectly (by reading his books and other writings). The prejudices which influenced British contemporaries did not affect the Americans. Reed's analysis of Tait's character also shows understanding and sensitivity:

> It were easy and natural in speaking of Mr. Tait to use such words as able, energetic, aggressive, inventive, resourceful, brave and tender, but it is not so easy to portray the psychic play whereby these and other qualities were blended in varying degree to produce the character that he revealed under varying circumstances. We can only follow the advice of Locke, who said that "the actions of men are the best interpreters of their thought" . . . . If we are to interpret Mr. Tait's character by his actions, we are at once impressed that he was a man of great action . . . . Mr. Tait had his full share of ambition . . . he was anxious to place his name on the scroll: he was proud of his achievements and he was interested that the record should be written with truth and justice. . . .
>
> He was distinctly the man for the time. At his advent professional opinion, like a dear old lady, was drowsing in an arm chair. He heralded new things in thunder tones, poked the drowsy jade in the ribs and broke up the siesta. Of course there were angry protests, but they availed nothing, for he went on thundering and prodding until everybody was awakened. That was his life.

In the years following his death Tait was largely forgotten. With Birmingham (in 1911) once again the host for the Annual Meeting of the

British Medical Association, Jordan Lloyd (1854-1913), Professor of Surgery in Birmingham, delivered the surgical address. He made reference to three local surgeons – Langston Parker, Oliver Pemberton and Lawson Tait. Lloyd recalled how Tait had given the surgical address 21 years previously, and said of his predecessor: "As a surgeon he was a genius: justice has not yet been done to him and possibly never will be, for the part he took in that wonderful development of abdominal surgery which occurred in the last quarter of the nineteenth century".[13]

In 1922 Stewart McKay published his long biography of Tait. It was McKay's intention to "bring home to the present generation what my great master did for abdominal surgery."[14] The book is a mine of information concerning Tait's life and character. His contributions to surgery are given in great detail, with long digressions into the historical background. Tait's quarrel with Lister is discussed very fully. The account has been criticised as partisan, for McKay remained Tait's disciple for life, just as Tait always remained the faithful disciple of Simpson. McKay's opinions have already been quoted. While he saw so many virtues in Tait he recognised that the working of his mind was all too frequently conditioned by prejudice or by preconceived notions. He appreciated that this weakness had made him obstinate over many things. McKay explained Tait's intransigent attitude to Listerism and to vivisection by excessive prejudices which "solidified his opinion and made it impregnable to evidence." He saw Tait as "one to whom criticism was a constant stimulus and antagonism but an incentive to further endeavours." McKay's account does not seem to have revived interest in Tait. The *British Medical Journal* gave the biography a long review but thought it ill-balanced and lacking discrimination. Christopher Martin's memoir, from which we have already quoted, appeared in 1931. This small book gives a remarkably clear picture of Tait and summarises his career.[15] Martin was closely associated with Tait for about ten years and his judgements are probably amongst the most reliable available to us.

The centenary of Tait's birth in 1945 did not pass unnoticed in Birmingham, but the celebrations were perhaps less elaborate than they might have been because of the War. The University, the Midland Medical Society and the Women's Hospital combined to arrange a ceremony at which the L.L.D. was conferred on Mr. Eardley Holland, President of the Royal College of Obstetricians and Gynaecologists, and on Major-General Hawley, Chief Surgeon to the American forces in Europe. The choices were appropriate, acknowledging Tait's place in the history of gynaecology and his influence on American surgery. An oration was delivered by Leonard Gamgee (1869-1956), son of Sampson Gamgee. Leonard Gamgee had attended Tait's lectures as a student.[16] He gave Tait credit for the establishment of aseptic surgery and described him as "the Napoleon of surgery—clear thinking, courageous, inventive, not bound by any precedent . . . He dispersed once and for all the fear and trepidation with which surgeons before his day opened the peritoneal cavity. He simplified abdominal surgery." The occasion aroused some interest and a few letters appeared in the local press with anecdotes of Tait's life.[17] A retired railwayman remembered him vividly as a frequent passenger well known to all the porters and guards on the Birmingham lines and remarkable for the amount of snuff he consumed. A clergyman wrote to describe how as a boy he had seen a rather corpulent and unhealthy Tait on the platform at a school prize-giving and recalled how Tait had munched biscuits untidily and noisily throughout the ceremony!

Seymour Barling (1880-1960), a nephew of the Gilbert Barling who had operated on Tait, wrote a centenary tribute in the *British Journal of Surgery.*[18] He described how Tait "had exercised immense influence when surgery was temporarily held back by the forces of tradition and conservatism." He appreciated, as had the American Charles Reed, that "something explosive was required to remove old prejudices towards the surgery of the abdomen." Of Tait's antagonism to Lister, he wrote that "Lister's work he neither understood or appreciated. He had found a method that suited him and sufficed. His success was empirical . . . . By chance he had taken a short cut which led to aseptic surgery." The *British Medical Journal* referred briefly to Tait's career in a leader entitled "A Great Abdominal Surgeon".[19] The *Lancet,* in reporting the Birmingham celebrations, attempted to define genius in surgery as a quality "often associated with an abundant and thirsty energy—an ability to do twice as much as anybody else in half the time." Tait certainly seemed to qualify as a genius under such a definition!

If in the 75 years since Tait died, doubt has remained concerning his true place in surgical history; his personality and character have continued to intrigue many writers. J. S. Tomkinson, for example, spoke in 1955 of him as a neglected figure in surgical history.[20] Sir Zachary Cope suggested in 1959 that Tait's contribution to surgery was little known because his quarrelsome nature and his opposition to Lister had made him many enemies. Cope accepted the idea that Tait had demonstrated the merits of asepsis over those of antisepsis.[21] Claud Taylor in 1965, chose for a Simpson Oration to the Royal College of Obstetricians and

Gynaecologists, "Lawson Tait – A grateful Pupil of James Young Simpson."[22] B.T.Davis has written with particular emphasis on Tait's activities in Birmingham.[23] A new biography written by Harvey Flack in 1948 was derived largely from the writings of McKay and Martin.[24] It is a balanced assessment of Tait's character and of his place as a surgical pioneer, with perhaps most emphasis (as with McKay) on Tait's gynaecological work. A memoir of Tait was written by Wilfred Risdon for the National Anti-Vivisection Society in 1967. As the author did not acquire a copy of McKay's biography, this account is somewhat deficient.[25]

If we attempt a modern appraisal of Tait's place in the history of surgery and gynaecology we may approach this in different ways. The new operations he devised may be listed and their survival (or otherwise) may be noted. It has already been emphasised that a "first" in itself is not particularly important, but that we should be more interested in the success of an individual in persuading others to adopt a new technique or to accept a new idea. We must assess the general influences exerted on surgery, influences which we now may see as having accelerated the progress of the art. We may compare Tait with other surgeons of his time who are recognised as pioneers or leaders.

Tait was the first to operate successfully for ruptured tubal pregnancy, and by his teaching he established the absolute necessity for this lifesaving procedure. His views on this remain unchallenged. His priority with regard to many of the other operations which he developed for diseases of the uterine appendages may be uncertain, but his establishment of the principles shown by these procedures cannot be questioned. He modified and improved many established gynaecological procedures, such as ovariotomy and perineal repair, but admitted that he was building on the experience of others. In ovariotomy his popularisation of the short ligature on the pedicle undoubtedly influenced the development of general abdominal surgery.

We have recorded how Tait was the first surgeon in the world to diagnose and remove successfully an acutely inflamed appendix. As he did not increase his experience of this condition, working as he did in a restricted field, he failed to persuade others to act on this new concept. Nevertheless he deserves a place in the history of the management of this very common acute abdominal emergency. In the surgery of the gallbladder and kidney Tait cannot be given priority for the introduction of the operations of cholecystostomy and nephrectomy, but his influence in advancing biliary and renal surgery in his own country was very great.

The new operations and the important modifications of existing procedures which Tait introduced might in themselves seem sufficient to establish him as a great surgeon. His more important contribution was, however, in his teaching of new principles in abdominal surgery. Over a period of less than 20 years Tait preached his new ideas to his colleagues repeatedly, forcibly, and even vehemently. The ultimate acceptance of his views must be seen as one of incalculable benefit in terms of relief of suffering and saving of human life.

We may summarise the important principles which Tait advanced. The first was that if a diseased condition was diagnosed with reasonable certainty and was amenable to surgery, then operation should not be delayed until symptoms became intolerable or acute. The second principle was that abdominal section (or laparotomy) should be employed freely as a diagnostic procedure. The third was that urgent operation should be done for acute complications of abdominal disease. The fourth was that there should be no fear of operating urgently for conditions associated with acute peritoneal infection. All these hold firmly today, and it is on just such principles that we base our present practice in elective and emergency abdominal surgery.

Tait propagated his original views in every possible way. His writings had considerable impact. His powerful style in debate – blustering, rude and sparing no adversary – was highly effective. If some of his arguments were at times deficient in logic and lacking in the application of scientific method, and if his statistics were at times careless, he was fundamentally honest concerning his results and he certainly convinced the general practitioners and his patients that he was right. Perhaps he made his points most effectively by direct teaching to his assistants and pupils, who came from all over the world to Birmingham to see his work.

While most of Tait's ideas were sound and have stood the test of time, it was inevitable that there were lapses. He persisted in his obscure tubal theory of menstruation all his life and was blind to proven facts which did not suit his explanations. His long advocacy of removal of the appendages to influence the growth and symptoms of fibroid tumours of the uterus is more excusable, for the operation was based on observed natural phenomena. His reluctance to perform hysterectomy for the eradication of large uterine tumours is difficult to explain, for he cannot be said to have lacked courage in dealing with technical difficulties in other operations. Tait is particularly faulted for his antagonism towards Lister. We must agree that in this he showed both obstinacy and a prejudice which blinded him to reason. Barling's assessment in this matter is astute and may be accepted. Tait evolved his own method for the safe performance of abdominal surgery by observing basic cleanliness and regulating the environment in which he worked. Having done so, he discovered that he could discard the details of the antiseptic system. From his particular experience in one field of surgery he was, however, wrong to generalise in the manner he did.

Two important questions arise over Tait's lifelong battle with Lister. Did he by his stormy interventions confuse the issues and so delay the development of safe surgery? Did he really play a part in the evolution of aseptic surgery? To the first question we may reply that there was more good than harm in Tait's role as devil's advocate. The criticisms he advanced, even though they were bigoted and unscientific, helped to clear the air. As to the second question, the answer is less certain. It is impossible to credit one man with the introduction of aseptic surgery, but we can agree with others that Tait exerted a considerable influence in the evolution of this technique.

Comparisons of Tait with other surgeons of his time are not easy to make. All accounts of the history of British surgery in the second half of the 19th century are dominated by the figure of Joseph Lister. His contribution was unique and came at a time when it was most needed. His discovery swept away the terrible consequences of hospital overcrowding, lack of hygiene, and the excessive operating which was the result of the introduction of general anaesthesia. He showed through his antiseptic system where lay the risks of wound infection. Others, including Tait, capitalised on this knowledge. Lister's fame is measured very largely on this work, and in terms of the saving of human life his achievement was immense. He must also be credited with the development of a scientific approach to surgery, although Sir James Paget deserves considerable recognition also for this advance. Neither Tait nor any other surgeon can be easily compared with Lister, for the general impact of his work rates with that of the discovery of general anaesthesia and, in more recent times, with that of the introduction of antibiotics. In intellect and genius, all other contemporary surgeons are overshadowed by Joseph Lister.

Tait may be compared more profitably with Spencer Wells, who was a pioneer in the same special field of surgery. Wells belonged to an earlier generation and his main expertise was in ovariotomy. He did operate on patients with uterine tumours, but relatively rarely did he undertake other abdominal procedures. By the time Tait came on the scene, Wells had made his main contribution by establishing ovariotomy as an acceptable and reasonably safe procedure. Tait soon outstripped Wells in his total experience. Between 1857 and 1880 Wells completed 1,000 ovariotomies. In 20 years, between about 1870 and 1890, Tait can be credited with some 5,000 abdominal operations of which approximately a quarter were ovariotomies, the remainder including a wide range of other abdominal procedures. Each contributed in a different way, but it was Tait who showed how the experience of the ovariotomists could be utilised to expand abdominal surgery.

Between 1870 and 1890 no British contemporary other than Spencer Wells even approaches Tait in the sheer volume of his experience in abdominal surgery; nor does anyone rival him in respect of the new operations he devised, the modifications of existing procedures which he introduced, or the range of new principles he popularised. His contribution to gynaecology has been given some recognition; however, his *total* contribution to surgery has been underestimated.

By now the reader must have appreciated the complexities of Lawson Tait's personality. The assessments of various contemporary observers have been recorded. After an interval of 75 years a biographer must depend greatly on the statements of others in making his own judgement. Samuel Johnson wrote of biographers that "they only who live with a man, can write his life with any genuine exactness and discrimination; and few people who have lived with a man know what to remark about him." The statement must not deter the biographer unduly! Posthumous psychological analysis is an exercise all too frequently indulged in by modern biographers (whether qualified professionally to attempt this or not). The temptation to indulge in this must be resisted because psychoanalysis cannot be undertaken on a dead man. But we do have our subject's writings, some surviving letters and his portraits to assist us in a reappraisal. We can, however, justifiably take into account some of the early influences which moulded his character.

Lawson Tait was of humble origin. He must soon have become aware of the opportunities given to the more privileged, compared to those offered to one who started life without social advantage. He was spurred on by his driving ambition, his enthusiasm and his readiness to work hard. He came up the hard way and it is not surprising that at times there was some uncertainty with regard to his social and professional position. This could be reflected by a degree of aggressiveness towards more favoured colleagues. There may well have been also the lack of confidence of a youthful expatriate, so often concealed by a superficial veneer or egoism and bravado. Not least he found himself involved in the traditional conflict between the provincial and the London surgeon. He must be seen against the mid-Victorian background, both scientific and social. His quick intelligence, his intense curiosity, his scepticism, and the rapidity with which he seized on new knowledge and philosophies made him, as Reed so clearly saw, "the man for the time." Most of his contemporaries, in contrast, supported established and orthodox opinions and distrusted any brash young man who defied convention. He was ahead of his time in so many matters, both in his social and professional activities. This is shown by his advanced views on such topics as medical education, the place of the woman doctor, sex education, religion and the application of Darwinism to human genetics and human activities. In Tait's time it was unusual, and indeed rash, for a young man to pit himself against his seniors, and he was probably perfectly aware that for the sake of his career it would have been wiser to conform. Tait was a rebel, but by his strong sense of conviction in so many matters he fought his way to a position of national and international importance. If often he was undiplomatic, uncompromising, cantankerous and rude in pressing his case, we must, however unhappily, accept the reality that peaceful persuasion would not have got him anywhere. When, after his long struggle, he was just beginning to be recognised for his ability and influence, everything went wrong. If his apparent failure was partly of his own making, we must surely be sympathetic and grant that it was a bitter judgement on him. Behind an exterior so often belligerent and obstinate there was a very human individual capable of charming all with whom he came in contact. He cared not only for his patients, but for all men and women. He was loyal to his friends and was always prepared to help the oppressed.

Of his intellect and his right to be considered a genius, it is less easy to judge. In all his activities he showed a remarkable ability and industry in collecting facts and mastering problems. At times he came to dogmatic conclusions too quickly and did not easily change his opinions. To support his claims he tended to bludgeon the opposition, for he was always in a hurry to have his ideas accepted. In his arguments he was not always logical. As was shown in his brief sally into botanical experiment, he was inadequately equipped as an experimental scientist.

Few influenced the specialty of surgery so markedly in such a short period of time as did Lawson Tait. Few have succeeded in cramming into their lives (and in Tait's case, such a short life) so much productive activity. It could be said that he attempted too much and that he could have achieved more if he had concentrated his remarkable energy on fewer subjects, but this simply was not his nature. It is not for us to sit in judgement on his morals, as did his contemporaries, to the detriment of his professional reputation. Let us be more generous and accord him a due place in the history of surgery. Let us remember him also as one of the outstanding and colourful personalities among the giants of the Victorian Age.

NOTES TO TEXT

Use has been made of numerous standard histories of medicine and surgery but I have not thought it necessary to list these. Tait was a great letter writer, but surprisingly few of his letters seem to have survived, with the exception of the Darwin series. It would seem that after his death his papers, which must have included many letters to him, were destroyed.

Where major quotations are given from any source, including Tait's writings, the appropriate reference is given. I have provided separately a bibliography with the titles of Tait's published letters, articles, pamphlets and books. These can be referred to very readily by date where there is comment upon them in the text.

CHAPTER I

1. McKay, W.S. (1922) "Lawson Tait: His Life and Work". Balliere, Tindall and Cox, London.

2. Recorded also in Martin, C. (1931) "Lawson Tait. The Man and his Work". Birmingham.

3. Records of George Heriot's School.

4. There is an illustration of the tombstone of Mrs. Tait in Martin (Ref. 2).

5. On Lawson Tait's marriage certificate his father's rank or profession is recorded as "gentleman".

6. Steven, E. (1845) "History of Heriot's Hospital" (revised 1859), Edinburgh. Also records of George Heriot's School.

7. For the background of medical teaching in Edinburgh and for details of the personalities of the time reference has been made freely to the invaluable Comrie, J.D. (1932) "History of Scottish Medicine". (Vol. 11), Wellcome Publications, Baillere, Tindall and Cox, London. The history of the Extramural School is to be found in Guthrie, D. (1965) "Extramural Medical Education in Edinburgh". Livingstone, Edinburgh.

8. Shepherd, J.A. (1970) "Simpson and Syme of Edinburgh". Livingstone, Edinburgh.

9. Simpson, J.Y. (1864) "Acupressure. A New Method of Arresting Surgical Haemorrhage and of Accelerating the Healing of Wounds". Black, Edinburgh.

10. This was almost certainly Arthur Gamgee (1841-1909), son of Joseph Gamgee and brother of Sampson Gamgee, the Birmingham surgeon. Arthur Gamgee graduated in Edinburgh and taught for a while in the Veterinary School as a lecturer in chemistry. For a full account of the Gamgees the reader is referred to Thompson, R.D. (1974) "The Remarkable Gamgees", Ramsay Head Press, Edinburgh.

11. Autobiography (unpublished) of McKay. I am indebted to Sir Edward Ford of Melbourne, Australia, for photostats of extracts from the manuscript.

12. These matters are recorded fully in the writer's "Simpson and Syme of Edinburgh". (Ref. 8). "Stories of the Temple", by "an Acolyte" (1862, Vickers, London) was suppressed at publication, but a few copies survive, including one in the Edinburgh City Library and one in the library of the Royal College of Surgeons of Edinburgh.

13. Many of Simpson's letters are held in the Library of the Royal College of Surgeons of Edinburgh and have recently been indexed by the Honorary Librarian Mr. J. Simpson Hall.

14. In 1885 when Tait gave a lecture to the class of Midwifery in Edinburgh, at the invitation of Sir Alexander Simpson, he is reported to have said "I cannot stand here, as it were in the shoes of my dead master, without feelings of emotion almost overwhelming me". (Edin. Med. J. 1886, 31, 812.)

15. Brit. Med. J. 1899, 1, 879.

16. Gray, J. (1952) "History of the Royal Medical Society, 1737-1937". University Press, Edinburgh.

17. The records of the Hunterian Society are in the Edinburgh University Library and include the Minutes during Tait's membership and copies of the "Laws of the Hunterian Medical Society of Edinburgh, 1868".

18. Brit. Med. J. 1887, 2, 166.

19. Brit. Med. J. 1890, 2, 267.

20. Geison, G. (1972) "Social and Institutional Factors in the Stagnancy of English Physiology 1840-1970". Bull. Hist. Med., 46, 30.

21. Some of Tait's certificates and diplomata survive. From these we know that he attended Simpson's obstetric course in 1863 and Goodsir's lectures on Comparative Anatomy in 1862. His College diplomata on final qualification are signed by James Dunsmore, P.R.C.S.E. and John Smith, P.R.C.P.E.

22. Ed. Med. J. 1881, 27, 864.

CHAPTER II

1. Med. Times and Gaz. 1867, 2, 24.

2. Annual Report of the Clayton Hospital and Wakefield Dispensary (1869). Further information from contemporary Medical Directories and from a collection of pamphlets and newspaper cuttings is in the Wakefield City Library.

3. "Sanitary Conditions of Wakefield". (Abstract). Med. Times and Gaz. 1870, 1, 36.

4. Syme, J. (1861) "Observations in Clinical Surgery". Edinburgh.

5. Lancet 1867, 1, 326.

6. Brit. Med. J. 1868, 1, 1.

7. This topic is discussed more fully in Shepherd, J.A. (1970) "Simpson and Syme of Edinburgh". Livingstone. Edinburgh.

8. Brit. Med. J. 1887, 2, 166.

9. Birm. Med. Rev. 1890, 27, 26.

10. Lancet 1866, 2, 254.

11. Dublin Quart. J. of Med. 1869, 47, 102.

12. There is a full description of Westgate House in a paper by Maxwell Reader (Practitioner 1971, 206, 691). Dr. O'Brien, the present occupant, kindly showed me the house and the loft which was Tait's simple laboratory.

13. Viets, H.R. (1938) "Crichton Browne 1840-1938". Bull. of Inst. of Hist. Med. 6, 472.

14. Tait's Fellowship diploma is extant and dated June 27th 1870. It is signed by James Gillespie, P.R.C.S.E. At this time the diploma was awarded after recommendation and no examination was taken.

CHAPTER III

1. Langford, J.R. (1873) "Modern Birmingham and its Institutions" (Vol. 1). Birmingham.

2. History of Birmingham School of Medicine". (anon.), 1925, Birmingham, and Vincent, E.W. and Hudson, P. (1947) "The University of Birmingham". Birmingham.

3. I am indebted to Dr. Gough of Birmingham for a historical note prepared by him for the Centenary celebrations of the foundation of the Women's Hospital.

4. Brit. Med. J. 1873, 2, 563 and 622.

5. Ibid. 1871, 2, 127, 185 and 219.

6. For a full account of the history of ovariotomy see Shepherd, J.A. (1965) "Spencer Wells". (Chap. 4). Livingstone, Edinburgh.

7. The Hastings Prize was established in 1860 for an essay by a member of the B.M.A. on some subject connected with the practice of medicine. The first gold medal was awarded to Dr. Thudicum in 1864, Mr. Furneaux Jordan of Birmingham gained the award in 1866, and Dr. Fothergill in 1870. Tait was the last to win this elegant medal, for the prize was discontinued in 1877. Tait's medal survives and is in private ownership.

8. Tait, R.L. (1883) "The Pathology and Treatment of Diseases of the Ovaries", p. 91. Birmingham.

9. The marriage took place on June 28th, 1871 in the Parish Church of Wakefield "according to the rites and ceremonies of the Established Church". (Wakefield Register.)

CHAPTER IV

1. I am indebted to Dr. F.M. Forster of Melbourne for information about Dr. Tracy and for extracts from his diary. It is of interest that Tracy had a paper read for him in London by Spencer Wells entitled "Case of Ovarian Dropsy Operated on During an Attack of Acute Peritonitis" (Med. Chir. Trans. 1873, 56, 20). Thus Tracy preceded Tait in operating for ovarian conditions during an acute crisis of peritonitis, but it was Tait who established this advance.

2. Ed. Med. J. 1885, 31, 201.

3. Battey described his operation in Atlanta Med. Surg. J. 1872, 10, 321, and in Brit. Med. J. 1880, 1, 36.

4. Ed. Med. J. 1885, 31, 201.

5. Ibid.

6. Parry, J. (1876) "Extra Uterine Pregnancy". Philadelphia.

7. Tait, R. L. (1888) "Lectures on Ectopic Pregnancy and Pelvic Haematocele". Richardson. Leicester.

8. Ibid.

9. Brit. Med. J. 1883, 2, 1116.

CHAPTER V

1. Trans. Indiana State Med. Soc. 1868, 68.

2. Sims travelled much in Europe, as recorded in Sims, J.M. (1885), "Story of My Life". New York. Tait came to know him well and dedicated one of his books, "Dear Dr. Marion Sims, I dedicate this volume to you as a token of the value I place on your friendship, and as an acknowledgement that much of the new work described in it is the outcome of your ingenuity, yours truly, Lawson Tait".

3. British Med. J. 1878, 1, 811.

4. Erichsen announced in his Address on Surgery at the Annual Meeting of the B.M.A. in Birmingham in 1886, "that the final limits in surgery have been reached in the direction of all that is manipulation and mechanical. . . . . we have reached finality in the mere mechanical art of surgery. Brit. Med. J. 1886, 2, 314.

5. Birm. Med. Rev. 1881, 16, 343.

6. For an account of the history of appendicitis see Shepherd, J.A. (1954) "Acute Appendicitis. A Historical Survey". Lancet 2, 298.

7. Birm. Med. Rev. 1890, 27, 26, and Lancet 1956, 2, 1301.

8. Ibid.

9. Trans. Path. Soc. 1868, 19, 295. (See also Ref. 1, Chap. IV)

10. Tait, R.L. (1883) "The Pathology and Treatment of Diseases of the Ovaries". (P. 323). Birmingham.

CHAPTER VI

(In the preparation of this chapter frequent reference has been made to the "Collected Writings of Lord Lister", "The Life of Lord Lister" by Rickman Godlee and "Antiseptic Surgery" by Watson Cheyne. Many biographies of Lister and Pasteur have been consulted and "The History of Bacteriology" by W. Bulloch has been useful. The papers given at the annual meetings of the B.M.A., to which frequent references are made, are to be found in the August issues of the British Medical Journal. The writings on the antiseptic system are in great quantity and I have limited references to those of basic importance and those bearing on the arguments which I have tried to develop on these controversial issues.)

1. Charles Darwin conceived his theories of evolution in his early life but the long period of gestation before he produced the "Origin of Species" was, in part, related to a conflict in his mind concerning the implications of his ideas on established Christian belief. See a recent study by Gruber, H.E. (1974) entitled "Darwin on Man". Welwood House. London.

2. My assessment of Lawrence may be a little harsh for Chance (1926), "Sir William Lawrence", Med. Hist. 8, 270, gives Lawrence considerable credit for the advance of ophthalmological surgery in his time.

3. "Life and Correspondence of Andrew Combe, M.D.". 1850. Edinburgh.

4. Mss in Edinburgh University Library (Gen. 580 D). This is the record, by an unknown student, of Goodsir's lectures. Tait's certificate of attendance at Goodsir's lectures still survives.

5. "Father and Son" by Edmund Gosse, was first published in 1907.

6. For a full account of Frascatorius (or Fracastoro) see Singer, C. and Singer, D. (1917) "The Scientific Position of Girolamo Fracastoro". Ann. Med. Hist. 1, 1.

7. Brit. Med. J. 1861, 2, 52.

8. Brit. Med. J. 1862, 2, 92.

9. Brit. Med. J. 1862, 2, 39 and 92. In the standard medical histories I can find only one writer, Mettler, who comments on Trousseau's grasp of the germ theory of disease.

10. Brit. Med. J. 1864, 2, 384.

11. Edin. Med. J. 1867-68, 13, 810.

12. Mss in Library of R.C.S. England.

13. Dawson, P.M. (1922) "Semmelweiss. An Interpretation". Ann. Med. Hist. 6, 258.

14. Lancet, 1867, 1, 326 and 357.

15. See Schecter, D.C. and Swan, H. (1961) "Jules Lemaire, a Forgotten Hero of Surgery". Surgery, 49, 817. Watson Cheyne (1882) "Antiseptic Surgery", London, was aware of his contribution and paid tribute to Lemaire in the first Lister memorial lecture in 1925 as amongst the first to appreciate the surgical

significance of Pasteur's discoveries. In the Edinburgh University Library there is a copy of the second edition of Lemaire, J. (1865) "L'Acide Phénique", Paris, most likely the copy Simpson and Lister consulted.

16. Lancet 1867, 2, 546.
17. Ibid. 1867, 2, 595.
18. Ibid. 1867, 2, 444 and 502.
19. Mss in Library of R.C.S. England.
20. Singer, C. (1928) "A Short History of Medicine". Oxford.
21. Brit. Med. J. 1867, 2, 246.
22. Mss in Wellcome Collection, London.
23. Brit. Med. J. 1869, 2, 143.
24. Ibid. 1869, 2, 256.
25. Ibid. 1871, 2, 225.
26. Ibid. 1879, 2, 210.
27. Lancet 1875, 2, 565.
28. Brit. Med. J. 1867, 2, 174.
29. It should be noted that many of the abscesses which Lister treated were the "cold" abscesses of tubercular disease. These were infected with tubercule bacilli but this organism was not at the time identified. Lister was correct in that these particular abscesses did not become infected with secondary pyogenic organisms until drained.
30. See Sherrington, C.S. (1927) "Lister as a Physiologist". Brit. Med. J. 1, 653; also Bulloch, "Lister as a Pathologist and Bacteriologist". Brit. Med. J. 1, 654.
31. Edin. Med. J. 1868-69, 14, 982.
32. Lancet 1875, 2, 597.
33. Farley, J. and Geison, C.G. (1974) "Science, Politics and Spontaneous Generation in Nineteenth Century France: the Pasteur-Pouchet debate". Bull. Hist. Med. 48, 161.
34. Brit. Med. J. 1887, 2, 161.
35. Enquiries from authorities ranging from professors of zoology to practical poultry keepers have given no confirmation of Tait's observation!
36. Brit. Med. J. 1891, 1, 381.
37. Brit. Med. J. 1890, 2, 377.
38. Brit. Med. J. 1890, 2, 728.
39. Brit. Med. J. 1882, 2, 830.
40. Lancet 1881, 2, 863 and 901.
41. Brit. Med. J. 1885, 1, 214.
42. Lancet 1891, 2, 597.

CHAPTER VI

(The letters quoted in this chapter are from three sources. Firstly, from the collection in the Library of Cambridge University, which includes most of Tait's letters to Charles Darwin. Secondly, there is in Shrewsbury School a small collection of Darwin letters including some to Tait. Thirdly, I have been fortunate in tracing some letters from Darwin to Tait which are in private ownership. The letters at Shrewsbury were given to the School by Mr. Stewart, a son of Tait's brother-in-law, and have been published in an article by Sir Gavin de Beer "The Darwin

Letters at Shrewsbury School" (Notes and Records Roy. Soc. Lond. 1963, 23, 68). After Darwin died his son borrowed from various individuals who had corresponded with his father as many letters as could be traced. A selection of these was published in "Letters of Charles Darwin" (1887), and a further selection in "More letters of Charles Darwin" (1903). Lawson Tait apparently lent his letters and two are quoted in the second collection. The letters were probably returned to Tait and when he died they were in the possession of the Stewart family and then rediscovered by me.

In the text the source of each letter quoted is indicated as follows:

a) Cambridge
b) Shrewsbury
c) Private ownership

1. The intensity of feeling against Darwinism is indicated by a newspaper report of Huxley's Edinburgh lecture. "The audience applauded this anti-scriptural and most debasing theory . . . . standing in blasphemous contradiction to biblical narrative and doctrine, instead of expressing resentment at the foul outrage committed upon them individually, and upon the whole species as made in the likeness of God by deserting the hall in a body, or using some more emphatic form of protest against the corruption of youth by the vilest and beastliest paradox ever invented in ancient or modern times by Pagan or Christian". (From "The Witness" of Jan. 11th, 1862, quoted by Atkins, H. (1974) "Down: The Home of the Darwins". Curwen Press.)

2. In Darwin, C.R. (1871), p. 168, Tait's paper is referred to very briefly in a footnote. Tait made the most of this somewhat sparse notice!

3. "Memoirs and Letters of Sir James Paget" (1901). Ed. by Stephen Paget. London.

4. Brit. Med. J. 1861, 2, 428.

5. In Turner, A.L. (1919) "Sir William Turner", Edinburgh, several letters from Darwin to Turner are quoted in full.

6. See Tait, R.L. (1883) "The Pathology and Treatment of Diseases of the Ovaries" (p. 177) for his theory.

7. Tait's paper on the umbilical cord (see Tait's own bibliography below) is not very revealing although the whole question of spiral growth is one of great interest and significance. It is worth noting that J.Y. Simpson had also been intrigued by this phenomenon and had published a paper "On the Causes of the Spiral direction of the Umbilical Vessels and Convolutions of the Cord in the Human Foetus". Ed. Med. J. 1859-60, 5, 22.

8. For a description of the ménage at Down House see Atkins, H. (1974) "Down: The Home of the Darwins". I am greatly indebted to Sir Hedley Atkins for additional information. Down House is preserved as a Darwin Museum in the care of the Royal College of Surgeons of England.

9. Darwin, C.R. (1874) "Insectivorous Plants".

10. This paper may have been the one published in "Nature" in 1873. See Tait's bibliography below.

11. There is a long paper published by Tait in 1879 "Researches on the Digestive Principles of Plants" but this is largely a repeat of the results of his

experiments between 1874 and 1875. Although he continued to follow new literature on the subject there is no real evidence that Tait had gone on with any experimental work.

12. Davis, B.T. (1972) "Lawson Tait – Friend of Women". J. Women's Med. Fed., October, 142.

CHAPTER VIII

1. The houses comprising the Crescent, now demolished, were all that were completed of a noble architectural plan, begun in 1792, which might have rivalled Georgian Bath.

2. J. Amer. Med. Ass. 1892, 18, 77 and 99.

3. Amer. J. Obstet. 1885, 18, 672.

4. Obituary of McKay (Med. J. Austr. 1948), 1, 353; Forster, F. (1967) "Three Australian Medical Historians". Med. J. Austr., 2, 927.

5. Mss of McKay's unpublished autobiography (Chap. 1, n. 11).

6. Irving, L. (1967) "The Successors". London.

7. Obituaries of Christopher Martin (Lancet 1933, 1, 279 and Brit. Med. J. 1933, 1, 206 and 295).

8. Martin, C. (1931) "Lawson Tait. His Life and Work, with Personal Reminiscences" (reprinted from Birmingham Medical Review).

9. Bland-Sutton, J. (1930) "The Story of a Surgeon". London.

10. Young, F.B. (1938) "Dr. Bradley Remembers". London.

11. The novel is quoted in the obituary of Tait in the Birmingham Daily Gazette. I have not been able to trace a copy.

12. Holmes, O.W. (1887) "Our Hundred Days in Europe".

13. The house is illustrated in McKay's biography. It has long been demolished and the gardens built over.

14. J. Amer. Med. Ass. 1892, 18, 99.

15; In a small greenhouse in the garden of St. Petrock's, Llandudno (where Tait spent his last years), there is a luxuriant and productive vine which he may well have planted.

16. Bush, R. (1942) "Soft Fruit Growing". Penguin Books. London.

17. Tait's consultant appointment in Southampton was the subject of many leaders and letters in the contemporary medical press and he participated vigorously in the correspondence.

18. The sermon is reprinted in McKay's biography but does not appear to have attracted any notice in the local press at the time.

19. The contemporary Birmingham newspapers report fully Lawson Tait's participation in the election.

20. This composite group was commissioned by the College and the artist Hay was paid 250 guineas. The President at the time was Joseph Bell. Probably Tait subscribed to the painting and so was included as an active fellow.

21. Cope, Z. (1959) "The Royal College of Surgeons of England. A History". Bland. London. The detailed reports of these matters are in the contemporary numbers of the British Medical Journal.

22. Brit. Med. J. 1885, 1, 43 and Brit. Gyn. J. 1895, 1, 3.

23. Brit. Med. J. 1875, 1, 646.

24. Brit. Med. J. 1881, 2, 97.

25. Tait was attacked for these critical remarks in an editorial (Boston Med. and Surg. J. 1884, 2, 328). He made a qualified apology to Spencer Wells in a letter to the British Medical Journal.

26. Warren's skeleton survives but is now concealed in a cabinet. In his will he directed that his remains should be exposed to view for all time for the edification of future medical students.

27. Amer. J. Obstet. 1899, 40, 840.

28. These were the Union College, Albany and the University of St. Louis. He received also an M.D. from the University of the State of New York and was accustomed to record this after his name as "M.D. Neo-Ebor". His honorary diplomata have not been traced.

29. The Bradley case is fully recorded in Med. T. and Gaz. 1885, 2, 265 and did much to arouse interest in the medico-legal problems of practitioners.

30. Forbes, R. (1948) "Sixty Years of Medical Defence". London.

31. Tait published this paper in the Brit. Med. J. 1882, 1, 677 and there were numerous reprints in pamphlet form in various languages.

32. Brit. Med. J. 1882, 1, 718.

33. Brit. Med. J. 1892, 2, 817 and 907.

34. Tait wrote to the "Times" on October 12th and November 8th 1892. In the October letter he replied to an argument that Harvey owed to experimental work on animals his discovery of the circulation of the blood by affirming that it was Servetus who deserved priority in this discovery (a controversy which still rages!),

35, Brit. Med. J. 1892, 2, 1024.

36. Publications of the Lawson Tait Research Trust.

37. Information concerning the Imlach case has been derived mainly from a large dossier in the Library of the Liverpool Medical Institution. This contains pamphlets, newspaper cuttings and much other material. Amongst others Gemmel, A. (1957) "Some Incidents in Surgery of the Ovary", J. Obst. and Gynec. 65, 392, and Sir Norman Jeffcoate in his presidential address to the Liverpool Medical Institution (Annual Report of L.M.I. 1967), have discussed the case.

38. As late as 1890 Dr. Malone of Illinois expressed the misgivings of surgeons in Britain and the United States in a paper entitled "Abuse of Abdominal Section", reported briefly in Brit. Med. J. 1890, 2, 184. He stated: "Since Lawson Tait electrified the world by his wonderful successes emulators have become numerous everywhere. There is scarcely a hamlet in the U.S. today where may not be found at least one who has opened a woman's belly and created a tombstone to the memory of his daring".

39. Carter, W. and Paul, F. (1886), "Case of Nephrectomy". Liver. Med. Chir. J., 7, 196.

40. Brit. Med. J. 1886, 2, 1195.

41. Tait's part in the Imlach case aggravated his relations with Spencer Wells. Tait quoted Wells in Prov. Med. J. 1887, 6, 2 as having said: "Since the Liverpool business I have not done an operation of this sort. There is little satisfaction in doing an operation which one may be prosecuted for like a common criminal". Tait's reply was, "not all the outcry of men whom I regard as wholly prejudicial, and to a large extent woefully ignorant, nor the threat of actions for damages, nor

abusive articles in either medical or daily papers, can make me swerve from what I believe my duty alike to my profession and my race."

42. Brit. Med. J. 1890, 1, 68.
43. Brit. Med. J. 1884, 1, 142.
44. Am. J. Obstet. & Gyn. 1937, 33, 249.
45. Brit. Med. J. 1893, 1, 398.

CHAPTER IX

1. Martin, F. (1934) "Fifty Years of Medicine and Surgery". Chicago.
2. Minutes of Royal College of Surgeons of Edinburgh, 1890.
3. The Denholm case is recorded fully (Brit. Med. J. 1892, 1, 726). It gave rise to many editorial comments and letters in the medical journals. See also a letter from Christopher Martin (Med. Press 1892, 104, 356).
4. I possess a copy of this rare pamphlet formerly in the possession of Eve Simpson, daughter of Sir James Simpson. I have traced no other copy. The pamphlet is dated January 10th, 1895.
5. This paper (Prov. Med. J. 1894, 1, 226) was not received very favourably. Tait's disclosures of his experience as an examining surgeon for the Birmingham Police were thought to be rather sordid. It was typical of Tait, however, to publicise these difficult medico-legal problems, without considering his own reputation. Unfortunately this interest of his augmented the accusations of immorality directed at him.
6. Minutes of Council and of the Journal and Finance Committee of the B.M.A., Jan. 16th, 1895.
7. Obituaries (Lancet 1898, 1, 191, Brit. Med. J. 1898, 1, 176, and Medical Press 1898, 1, 45). There is further information concerning Dr. Hart in a history of the B.M.A., Vaughan, P. (1959) "Doctor's Commons". London.
8. Chesney, K. (1971) "Victorian Underworld". Victorian Book Club. Newton Abbot.
9. There is evidence in an American journal (N.Y. Med. J. 1895, 1, 178) that a comment on the Tait v. Hart case appeared in the "Sun" newspaper.
10. Dr. D.G. Boddington has kindly sent me some recollections of conversations with his grandfather Professor Gamgee.
11. Martin, C. (1931) "Lawson Tait". Birmingham.
12. Barling, G. (1931) "Reminiscences of Lawson Tait. Birm. Med. R. 6, 137.

CHAPTER X

1. Lancet 1898, 2, 159.
2. Brit. Med. J. 1897, 1, 1530.
3. Lancet 1897, 1, 1687.
4. The house still stands with only slight alterations since it was built. The site is an old quarry with, at the West side, the entrance to Gogarth's cave, screened by a large fig tree. From photographs taken in Tait's time the terraced garden seems relatively unchanged and is ingeniously planned. There is a simple inscription on an outer wall with the initials of Tait and his wife and the date of their first occupation of the house in May 1888.

5. Reports in "Landudno Advertiser", 1898-1899.

6. Reports in medical press, "Liverpool Daily Post", "Llandudno Advertiser" and the "Times".

7. Records in Anfield Crematorium with the note "disposal of ashes in private grounds".

8. Information of this inscription from the Lawson Tait Medical and Scientific Trust. The memorial stone cannot be traced and certainly is not now in St. Gogarth's cave.

9. B.M.J. 1899, 2, 381 and records in Somerset House.

CHAPTER XI

1. Birmingham Daily Gazette, June 14th, 1899.

2. Birmingham Post, June 14th, 1899.

3. Liverpool Daily Post, June 16th, 1899.

4. M.A.P. ("Mainly about People") 1899, June 24th. Birmingham.

5. Undated press cutting.

6. Brit. Med. J. 1899, 2, 1486.

7. Brit. Med. J. 1899, 2, 1561.

8. Lancet 1899, 2, 1736.

9. Med. Press 1899, 1, 656.

10. Trans. Obst. Soc. Lond. 1900, 42, 59. For another rather guarded tribute from a gynaecologist see also the Presidential Address to the British Gynaecological Society given by McNaughton-Jones (Brit. Gyn. J. 1899, 15, 546).

11. Practitioner 1899, 63, 4.

12. J.A.M.A. 1899, 33, 875. For a retrospective American tribute see also an editorial by J.H. Kellog who studied under Tait. (Surg. Gyn. Obst. 1930, 50, 914).

13. Brit. Med. J. 1911, 2, 206.

14. McKay, S. (1922) "Lawson Tait. His Life and Work". Bailliere, Tindall and Cox. London.

15. Martin, C. (1931) "Lawson Tait. His Life and Work, with Personal Reminiscences" (reprinted from Birmingham Medical Review). Martin published these reminiscences originally in J. Obst. Gyn. of B.E. 1921, 28, 117.

16. Surg. Gyn. Obstet. 1945, 52, 592.

17. Filed in Birmingham City Library.

18. Brit. J. Surg. 1945-46, 33, 80.

19. Lancet 1945, 2, 253.

20. Tomkinson, J.S. (1955) "Lawson Tait, Father of Abdominal Surgery". Guys Hosp. Gaz. 69, 371.

21. Cope, Z. (1959) "Lawson Tait". Central African J. Med. 5, 309.

22. Taylor, C.W. (1965) "Lawson Tait – A Grateful Pupil of James Young Simpson". J. of Obst. and Gyn. of Brit. Commonwealth, 72, 165.

23. Davis, B.T. (1922) "Lawson Tait – Friend of Women". J. Womens Med. Fed., October, 142.

24. Flack, I.H. (1949) "Lawson Tait 1845-1899". Heinemann. London.

25. Risdon, W. (1967) "Robert Lawson Tait". Murray, Edwards and Co. London. (Published by National Antivivisection Society)

BIBLIOGRAPHY OF LAWSON TAIT

This list has been prepared from a search of British and American medical and scientific journals. In checking against the references and bibliographies given by previous biographers there has been difficulty in confirming some attributions in American medical journals. It has not been possible to trace all Tait's writings in newspapers. References to "abstracts" of papers are included only if the full paper has not been traced. Like most of his contemporaries Tait circulated copies of many papers either as reprints or in pamphlets which might include additional material. I have included only those pamphlets for which I have failed to trace an original publication.

It has been thought worth recording Tait's literary output as completely as possible. The titles show his extraordinary industry, curiosity and versatility. His letters reveal his relentless criticism of his colleagues and of contemporary institutions, and his persistence in pressing his views. When it is realised that there are, in addition, very many contributions to medical societies in the form of case reports or presentations of pathological specimens it is astonishing that he found the time to present so much material. Admittedly there is much repetition in some of his papers but a total of 328 items, not counting 270 letters, covering a period of thirty-two years is remarkable. Sir James Simpson in a period of twenty-five years contributed 214 items to medical and scientific journals, and Sir Thomas Spencer Wells published 317 items over a period of forty-five years.*

It was unusual before 1900 for medical authors to contribute joint papers to the journals and books by joint authors were also relatively rare. On one occasion Tait collaborated with Christopher Martin in an article and there is an unconfirmed record of an article by him and the American gynaecologist Mundé in an American journal. But he was essentially an individualist!.

Tait's first contribution to the medical press was in 1863, a letter concerning a case he had observed as a student in the Edinburgh Royal Infirmary. His last contribution, not inappropriately, was a letter of protest in the British Medical Journal. Some American writers have

---

* These figures are necessarily approximate but are comparative.

suggested that his last publication was a paper, "The story of a sore kidney", an account of his own illness. In fact this was to be the subject of an address to a North Wales medical society in May 1899 but it was never delivered nor printed. There is a short paper attributed to him and published posthumously in "Amateur Gardening" in August, 1899, entitled "On bulb culture".

In the separate list of books and monographs there are ten items. We know of two other projected books which were never completed–the second volume of his "Diseases of Women and Abdominal Surgery" and a biography of Charles Clay. No manuscripts of these works have been discovered.

N.B. 270 letters written by Tait to the Journals are listed but the total is very much greater. Letters of a trivial or repetitive nature have been omitted.

I. EARLY MISCELLANEOUS PAMPHLETS.

Britain during the Stone Age.
Prehistoric fortifications.
Monumental brasses.
Kitchen middens and other prehistoric remains in Scotland.
The orientation of churches.

(These pamphlets are reprints from Wakefield newspapers; the exact dates are uncertain.)

II. JOURNAL ARTICLES

1863

–Medical Times and Gazette.
A remarkable case of apoplexy (letter). 1863, 1, 101.

1864

–Edinburgh Medical Journal.
Case of abortion of twins (abstract). 1863-64, 9, 93.

1865

–Med. T. and G.
Acupressure – experiments on lower animals (letter). 1865, 1, 502.
On the results of temporary metallic compression of arteries. 1865, 2, 57, 85.
The employment of paraffine in the construction of an apparatus immobile for fractures (letter). 1865, 2, 714.

1866

–Med. T. and G.
On the treatment of fracture of the radius at the styloid process by means of Gordon's splint. 1866, 1, 170.
Note on acupressure. 1866, 1, 197.
Notes of some cases in which acupressure was employed. 1866, 1, 335.
Fracture of the radius at the styloid process (letter). 1866, 1, 349.
Paraffin. 1866, 2, 471.

1867

–Med. T. and G.
Note on Acupressure. 1867, 1, 332.
An easy method of taking casts. 1867, 2, 168.
Mr. Gant's pathological surgery of the arteries. 1867, 2, 417.
On the treatment of femoral aneurysm. 1867, 2, 534.
–Ed. Med. J.
Colles Fracture. 1866-7, 12, 904.
Notes on preparation jars. 1866-7, 12, 1107.
–Science Gossip.
On tape worms in birds. 1867, August.

1868

–Med. T. and G.

Metalbumen in the urine (letter). 1868, 1, 652.

Torsion versus acupressure. 1868, 2, 106.

Effects of carbolic acid. 1868, 2, 465.

–Ed. Med. J.

Cancer curing (letter). 1868-9, 14, 190.

–British Medical Journal.

A substitute for the ligature (letter). 1868, 1, 314.

–Lancet.

Tapeworm in birds (letters). 1868, 1, 145 and 214.

–Dublin Quart. Journal of Medicine.

Fractures of the thigh. 1868, 1, 70.

On chorea. 1868, 1, 203.

1869

–Med. T. and G.

Syphilitic hemiplegia from deposit in the nerve tissue and plugging of the arteries. 1869, 1, 219.

Aneurysm Compressor (letter). 1869, 1, 349.

The theory of development (letter). 1869, 1, 481.

Reduction of chronic inversion of the uterus (abstract). 1869, 2, 116.

Fungus of the Dura Mater. 1869, 2, 427.

The foot and mouth exanthem (letter). 1869, 2, 506.

–Ed. Med. J.

On oedema of the conjunctiva as a symptom of surgical fever. 1868-8, 14, 798.

Case of death from strangulated ovarian tumour. 1869-70, 15, 502.

–Brit. Med. J.

The theory of life (letter). 1869, 1, 362.

The action of mercury on the liver (letter). 1869, 2, 132.

–Lancet.

Ligature, acupressure and torsion (letter). 1869, 1, 695 and 805.

On the treatment of intermaxillary cleft (letter). 1869, 2, 290.

On a new method of using needles in the operation for harelip. 1869, 2, 435.

–Dubl. Quart. J. Med.

Notes on the abnormalities of serous membranes. 1869, 2, 85.

Has the law of natural selection by survival of the fittest failed in the case of man? 1869, 2, 102.

On the cure of uterine epilepsy. 1869, 2, 536.

–Journal of Anatomy and Physiology.

Notes on some peculiar tumours found on the Gasterosteus Tracturais (Stickleback). 1869, 4, 12.

Notes on unusual accessory muscles. 1869, 4, 236.

–Obstetrical Transactions (London).

Case of reduction of chronic inversion of the uterus by sustained pressure. 1869, 11, 174.

1870

–Med. T. and G.

Note on the foot and mouth exanthem – case where it was closely simulated in the human subject. 1870, 1, 93.

The action of chloral hydrate (letter). 1870, 1, 193.

Note on Stilling's operation for stricture of the lachrymal duct. 1870, 2, 421.

Labio-glosso-laryngeal paralysis. 1870, 2, 667.

–Brit. Med. J.

Case of complicated lithotomy successfully treated. 1870, 1, 458.

The rapid pressure treatment of aneurysm (letter). 1870, 2, 263.

The influence of milk in the propagation of contagious diseases. 1870, 2, 344.

–Lancet.

On the use of simple syrup as a collyrium. 1870, 1, 228.

Case of complicated lithotomy successfully treated. 1870, 1, 477.

The operation of extirpation of the coccyx (letters). 1870, 1, 714 and 2, 690.

On the treatment of tetanus by woorali, calabar bean, and chloral hydrate. 1870, 2, 466.

On the cure of the chronic perforating ulcer of the bladder by the formation of an artificial vesico-vaginal fistula. 1870, 2, 738.

–British and Foreign Medico-Surgical Review.

On the variety of periosteal disease generally known as fungus of the dura mater. 1870, 45, 196.

–Pamphlet.

Note on a method of administering ether vapour. 1870.

1871

–Med. T. and G.

Operations for vaginal fistulae. 1871, 1, 332.

On a case of encephaloid cancer of the femur treated by electrolysis (abstract). 1871, 1, 498.

–Brit. Med. J.

On the treatment of suppurating glands in the neck by frequently repeated tapping. 1871, 1, 117.

Tracheotomy in infants. 1871, 1, 391.

Medical experts in Courts of Law (letters). 1871, 2, 127 and 219.

–Lancet.

Cases treated antiseptically on Lister's method. 1871, 1, 45.

Mr. Holmes on "Hospitalism" (letters). 1871, 1, 139 and 159.

A consideration of the criticisms advanced on Sir Jas. Y. Simpson's papers on "Hospitalism" especially those of Mr. Holmes. 1871, 1, 443.

Strange course of a uterine sound (letter). 1871, 1, 594.

–Dubl. Quart. J. Med.

Laryngismus stridulus. 1871, 1, 116.

On the myoidema of phthisis. 1871, 2, 316.

–Brit. For. Med. Chir. R.

On the treatment of cleft palate. 1871, 46, 181.

–Nature.

A new view of Darwinism (letter). 1871, 4, 201.

1871 (cont'd.)

–Pamphlet.

Nursing by nurses. 1871. Birmingham.

1872

–Med. T. and G.

The declaration concerning alcohol (letter). 1872, 1, 88.

A new form of trochar for use in ovariotomy (abstract). 1872, 2, 638.

–Brit. Med. J.

Note on the cure of inveterate eczema in children by vaccination. 1872, 1, 92.

Statistics of ovariotomy (letter). 1872, 1, 581.

The treatment of inertia of the uterus. 1872, 1, 668.

Absence of the uterus after repeated pregnancies. 1872, 2, 465.

–Lancet.

Strange course of a uterine sound (letter). 1872, 1, 559.

Case of utero-peritoneal fistula. 1872, 1, 680.

Utero-peritoneal fistula. 1872, 2, 557.

–Birmingham Medical Review.

Extra-uterine therapeutics. 1872, 1, 283.

–Nature.

Cranial measurements. 1872, 5, 463.

–Pamphlet.

On the myoidema of phthisis. 1872. Birmingham.

1873

–Med. T. and G.

A successful case of gastrotomy in extra-uterine gestation (abstract). 1873. 1, 213.

On the diagnosis of extra-uterine pregnancy (abstract). 1873, 1, 561.

Death under the administration of methylene ether. 1873, 2, 3.

Case of extra-uterine foetation. 1873, 2, 119.

–Brit. Med. J.

Methylene ether (letter). 1873, 1, 353.

Sir James Simpson's schedules. 1873, 2, 589.

–Lancet.

Methylene ether (letter). 1873, 1, 225.

Extra-uterine foetation (letter). 1873, 1, 169.

–Medico-Chirurgical Transactions.

Successful case of gastrotomy in extra-uterine pregnancy. 1873, 56, 219.

–Nature.

Note on a polydactylous cat from Cookham Dean. 1873, 7, 323.

–Obstetric Journal of Great Britain and Ireland.

Menstrual irregularities and their relation to diseases of the nervous system. 1873, 1, 94 and 173.

1874

–Med. T. and G.

Note on sponge tents. 1874, 1, 35.

The galvanic stem (letter). 1874. 1, 443.

Case of successful removal of a large fibro-myoma of the fundus uteri by abdominal section (abstract). 1874, 2, 565.

–Brit. Med. J.

On the pathology and treatment of ovarian diseases (Hastings prize essay 1873). 1874, 1, 701, 733, 765, 798, 825, and 2, 8 and 29.

–Lancet.

Mr. Lawson Tait's staining fluid (letter). 1874, 1, 393.

Case of successful removal of a large fibro-myoma from the fundus uteri (letter). 1874, 2, 680.

–Obstet. Trans.

Note on the diagnosis of extra-uterine pregnancy. 1874, 15, 135.

–J. of Anat. and Phys.

On the freezing process for section cutting: and on various methods of staining and making slides. 1874, 9, 249.

–Birm. Med. R.

On the medical education of women. 1874, 3, 81.

1875

–Med. T. and G.

Cells in ovarian fluid (letters). 1875, 1, 428 and 535.

Congenital deficiency of the peritoneum resulting in intestinal obstruction, and simulating an abdominal tumour (abstract). 1875, 2, 137.

–Edin. Med. J.

Enlargement of the thyroid body in pregnancy. 1874-1875, 20, 993.

–Lancet.

Metro-peritoneal fistula in a case of successful ovariotomy. 1875, 1, 45.

Section cutters (letter). 1875, 2, 40.

The late Dr. Hughes Bennet (letter). 1875, 2, 509.

–Obst. Trans.

A case of general dropsy in a foetus. 1875, 17, 397.

Note on a diseased placenta. 1875, 17, 326.

–Birm. Med. R.

On puerperal endocarditis. 1875, 4, 101, 197 and 233.

–Nature.

Insectivorous plants. 1875, 12, 251.

1876

–Med. T. and G.

The proposed alterations of the laws of the British Medical Association (lerter). 1876, 2, 189.

1876 (cont'd.)

–Lancet.

Premature closure of foramen ovale (letter). 1876, 1, 302.

Saccular dilatation of the urethra (letter). 1876, 1, 763.

–Obst. Trans.

Case of vesico-vaginal fistula left fourteen years after lithotomy, cured by a series of plastic operations. 1876, 18, 209.

–Birm. Med. R.

Case of puerperal endocarditis. 1876, 5, 125.

–Proceedings of the Royal Society.

Preliminary note on the anatomy of the umbilical cord. 1876, 166, 417.

–Practitioner.

Nélaton's inversion method in a chloroform accident. 1876, 16, 102.

New method of administering ether vapour. 1876, 16, 207.

–Pamphlet.

The evolution of our moral life. 1876. Birmingham Gazette.

1877

–Med. T. and G.

Hospital mortality (letters). 1877, 2, 424 and 527.

–Brit. Med. J.

Statistics of hospital mortality (letter). 1877, 2, 609.

–Lancet.

The Fallacies of statistics (letter). 1877, 2, 181.

Hospital mortality (letters). 1877, 2, 260, 295, 334 and 410.

After-history of a case of ovariotomy. 1877, 2, 686.

–Obst. Trans.

Four cases of removal of large uterine myomata by abdominal section. 1877, 19, 274.

–Transactions Birmingham Natural History Society.

A criticism of the doctrine of individuality. 1877.

–Nature.

Gallion's whistles (letter). 1877, 15, 294.

–Pamphlet.

A letter on hospital mortality addressed to the Governors of Birmingham General Hospital. 1877. Birmingham.

1878

–Med. T. and G.

Treatment of chronic inversion of the uterus (abstract). 1878, 1, 602.

–Brit. Med. J.

Statistics of hospital mortality (letter). 1878, 2, 609.

Menstrual fluid retained in the left Fallopian tube and simulating ovarian tumour; abdominal section during acute peritonitis. 1878. 1, 677.

1878 (cont'd.)

(–Brit. Med. J.)

Case of retention of menstrual fluid in the Fallopian tube: a reply to Dr. Harley. 1878, 1, 933.

Two cases of removal of small ovarian tumours on account of uterine haemorrhage. 1878, 2, 596.

–Obst. Trans.

Two cases of repair of the female bladder and urethra. 1878, 20, 88.

–Nature.

Note on the occurrence of sacral dimple and its possible significance. 1878, 18, 481.

1879

–Med. T. and G.

Case of cholecystostomy performed for dropsy of the gall-bladder due to impaction by a stone (abstract). 1879, 2, 594.

On new methods of operation for repair of the female perineum (abstract). 1879, 2, 597.

–Brit. Med. J.

Removal of normal ovaries. 1879, 1, 613.

Oophorectomy performed successfully for menstrual epilepsy. 1879, 2, 730.

The parthenogenetic development of dermoid cysts of the ovary (letter). 1879, 2, 761.

A second successful case of gastrotomy in extra-uterine pregnancy (abstract). 1879, 2, 779.

Tait's knot. 1879, 2, 813.

The Staffordshire knot. 1879, 2, 1021.

–Lancet.

Case of successful removal of a parovarian cyst which had become gangrenous from rotation and strangulation of its pedicle. 1879, 1, 915.

Twelve cases in which dilatation of the cervix uteri was accomplished by continuous elastic pressure. 1879, 2, 668.

Use of continuous elastic pressure in surgical practice (letter). 1879, 2, 709.

–Obst. Trans.

On new methods of operation for repair of the female perineum. 1879, 21, 292.

–Trans. Birm. Nat. Hist. Soc.

Researches on the structure of pitcher plants. 1879.

–Birmingham Philosophical Society Transactions.

The evolution of the sense of hearing. 1879, 1, 83.

–Nature.

The uses of tails. 1879, 20, 603.

1880

–Med. T. and G.

The Listerian method in ovariotomy. 1880, 1, 689.

1880 (cont'd.)

(–Med. T. and G.)

The Listerian method in ovariotomy. A rejoinder. 1880, 2, 98.

An instance of the mischievous effect which may arise from the Listerian precautions in abdominal section. 1880, 2, 128.

–Brit. Med. J.

Dr. Chambers on oophorectomy (letter). 1880, 1, 154.

A third case of extra-uterine gestation treated by abdominal section (abstract). 1880, 1, 757.

Note on oophorectomy. 1888, 1, 48.

Oophorectomy in dysmennorrhoea (abstract). 1880, 1, 230.

The history of ovariotomy (letter). 1880, 1, 317.

Cure of menstrual epileptic mania treated by oophorectomy (abstract). 1880, 12, 379.

The Birmingham and Midland Eye Hospital (letter). 1880, 2, 530.

Case of hydatids of the liver treated by abdominal section and drainage (abstract). 1880, 2, 975.

Paraffin splints (letter). 1880, 2, 1006.

–Lancet.

The diagnosis of ovarian tumours from the characters of the fluids contained in them. 1880, 1, 205.

Lister's antiseptic dressings (letter). 1880, 1, 666.

A fifth case of extra-uterine pregnancy treated by abdominal section. 1880, 2, 456.

Chian turpentine in cancer (letters). 1880, 2, 595 and 675.

–Obst. Trans.

On axial rotation of ovarian tumours leading to their strangulation and gangrene. Three cases successfully treated by immediate ovariotomy. 1880, 22, 86.

–Med.-Chir. Trans.

Case of cholecystotomy performed for dropsy of the gall-bladder due to impaction of a gall-stone. 1880, 63, 17.

The antiseptic theory tested by the statistics of one hundred cases of successful ovariotomy. 1880, 63, 161.

On the treatment of pelvic suppuration by abdominal section and drainage. 1880, 63, 307.

–Birm. Med. R.

A case of exanthematic cirrhosis of the ovary. 1880, 9, 52.

–Birm. Phil. Soc. Trans.

Note on bedroom ventilation. 1880, 2, 151.

1881

–Med. T. and G.

Hydatids of the liver treated by abdominal section and drainage. 1881, 1, 51.

Ovariotomy and the late Mr. Baker Brown (letters). 1881, 1, 278 and 358.

Listerian details in ovariotomy (letter). 1881, 1, 659.

Three cases of hepatotomy (abstract). 1881, 1, 661.

1881 (cont'd.)

(–Med. T. and G.)

Removal of uterine appendages for the arrest of haemorrhage (abstract). 1881, 1, 661,

The discussion on "Battey's operation" (letter). 1881, 2, 371.

An account of one hundred and ten consecutive cases of abdominal section. 1881, 2, 544 and 625.

A case of removal of the uterine appendages for the arrest of haemorrhage.. 1881, 2, 654.

Fourteen specimens of hydro- and pyo-salpinx (abstract). 1881, 2, 752.

–Brit. Med. J.

Listerian ovariotomy (letters). 1881, 1, 29 and 320.

The classification of ovarian operations (letter). 1881, 1, 140.

A case of removal of the uterine appendages. 1881, 1, 766.

A case of hepatotomy for hydatids. 1881, 2, 81.

Recent advances in pelvic surgery (abstract). 1881, 2, 391.

The success of oophorectomy (letter). 1881, 2, 505.

The discussion on the treatment of intraperitoneal tumours at the Congress (letter). 1881, 2, 615.

Abdominal section as an aid to pathological investigation (letter). 1881, 2, 759.

Dilation and suppuration of the Fallopian tubes (abstract). 1881, 2, 938.

–Lancet.

"Listerian" ovariotomy (letter). 1881, 1, 35.

The Birmingham Hospital for Women (letters). 1881, 1, 518 and 558.

Case of removal of large cystoma of ovary, followed by disappearance of a uterine myoma. 1881, 1, 578.

Case of complete disappearance of a large uterine myoma within six months of removal of uterine appendages (letter). 1881, 2, 687.

–Birm. Med. R.

A series of fifty cases of abdominal section for various purposes. 1881, 10, 30.

Debate on the clinical results obtained by the Listerian methods of performing operations and dressing wounds. 1881, 10, 79.

Four cases of hepatotomy. 1881, 10, 343.

1882

–Med. T. and G.

On death after ovariotomy, due to previous tapping (abstract). 1882, 1, 267.

Note on two cases of abdominal section. 1882, 2, 74.

–Brit. Med. J.

An experimental research on the value of the details of Listerism in abdominal surgery (abstract). 1882, 1, 543.

The vivisection discussion (letters). 1882, 1, 558 and 718.

Simple and aseptic ovariotomy (letter). 1882, 1, 838.

Removal of the uterine appendages (letter). 1882, 2, 153.

1882 (cont'd.)

(–Brit. Med. J.)

Remarks on the diagnosis and treatment of chronic inflammation of the ovary. 1882, 2, 161.

Mr. Lawson Tait and Listerism (letter). 1882, 2, 341.

Death under ether (letter). 1882, 2, 103.

One hundred consecutive cases of ovariotomy performed without any of the Listerian details. 1882, 2, 830.

Telephones for zymotic hospitals (letter). 1882, 2, 924.

A successful case of nephrectomy. 1882, 2, 929.

A third successful case of cholecystotomy. 1882, 2, 990.

Extra-uterine pregnancy. 1882, 2, 1092.

Movable kidney (letter). 1882, 2, 1178.

Mr. Steele's case of extra-uterine pregnancy (letter). 1882, 2, 1232.

Parallel histories of two cases of bleeding myoma. 1882, 2, 1294.

–Lancet.

The operation of spaying in women (letters). 1882, 1, 1009

Death after abdominal operations from heart-clot, due to disease of the kidneys. 1882, 2, 889.

Death after abdominal operations from heart-clot, due to disease of the kidneys (letters). 1882, 2, 1004 and 1137.

–Birm. Med. R.

Two cases of hydatids of the peritoneum successfully treated by abdominal section. 1882, 11, 193.

–Birm. Phil. Soc. Trans.

On the uselessness of vivisection upon animals as a method of scientific research. 1882, 3, 121.

–Medical Press and Circular.

Mr. Lawson Tait as an antivivisectionist (letter). 1882, 1, 431.

A research into the value of the details of Lister's method in abdominal surgery. 1882, 1, 243.

–American Journal of Medical Science.

Removal of uterine appendages for the arrest of uterine haemorrhage. 1882, 83, 48.

1883

–Brit. Med. J.

Movable kidney (letter). 1883, 1, 182.

An account of two hundred and eight consecutive cases of abdominal section performed between Nov. 1st 1881 and December 31st 1882. 1883, 1, 300.

Pyosalpinx (letter). 1883, 2, 997.

On the radical cure of exomphalus. 1883, 2, 1118.

–Lancet.

Death after abdominal operations from heart-clot (letter). 1883, 1, 38.

Ovariotomy statistics (letters). 1883, 1, 122 and 520.

Length of incisions in ovariotomy. 1883, 2, 388.

1883 (cont'd.)

–Obst. Trans.

A note on uterine myoma, its pathology and treatment. 1883, 25, 294.

Three cases of pyosalpinx. 1883, 25, 234.

A case of idiopathic gangrene of the uterus. 1883, 25, 248.

An undescribed disease of the Fallopian tube. 1883, 25, 249.

–Nature.

The uselessness of vivisection (letter). 1883, 28, 589.

–Birm. Phil. Soc. Trans.

Notes on ventilation of public buildings. 1883, 3, 110.

Utilisation of town refuse, as illustrated by the process adopted by the Birmingham Corporation. 1883, 3, 447.

Delaney's synchronous multiplex telegraphy. 1883, 3, 484.

–Glasgow Medical Journal.

Malpositions of the kidney (letter). 1883, 20, 194.

1884

–Med. T. and G.

Note on the relations of ovulation and menstruation. 1884, 1, 619.

Hydro- and Pyo-Salpinx (letters). 1884, 1, 681, 815 and 881.

Sir Spencer Wells on early and late removal of abdominal tumours. 1884, 2, 66.

Case of intestines adherent behind uterus, causing intense pain, 1884, 2, 79.

Post-mortem examination of a case in which removal of the uterine appendages for myoma had been performed three years before death. 1884, 2, 147.

Removal of the uterine appendages for myoma (letter). 1884, 2, 235.

Hydro- Pyo and Haemato-Salpinx. 1884, 2, 319.

The revival of ovariotomy. 1884, 2, 763.

Notes on the causation of labour. 1884, 2, 776.

–Brit. Med. J.

Note on cholecystostomy. 1884, 1, 853.

Five cases of extra-uterine pregnancy operated upon at the time of rupture. 1884, 1, 1250.

Pneumonotomy (letter). 1884, 1, 1278.

Surgical treatment of gall-stone. 1884, 2, 67.

The pathology and treatment of extra-uterine pregnancy. 1884, 2, 317.

The revival of ovariotomy (letter). 1884, 2, 1165.

–Lancet.

Two instances of remarkable elevation of temperature. 1884, 2, 59.

–Birm. Med. R.

The surgery of the kidney. 1884, 16, 1.

American Notes. 1884, 16, 241.

–Nature.

Note on deafness in white cats. 1884, 29, 164.

–Am. J. Obst.

Listerism in abdominal surgery (letter). 1884, 17, 676.

1884 (cont'd.)

–Med. Press and C.

History of a case of chronic ovaritis four years after removal of the uterine appendages. 1884, 2, 70.

Note on removal of the uterine appendages for inflammatory disease. 1884, 2, 433.

Recent advances in pelvic surgery. 1884, 1, 321 and 347.

Case of suprapubic lithotomy in a woman – an exceptional case. 1884, 1, 558.

–New York Medical Journal.

A clinical lecture. 1884, 1, 421.

1885

–Med. T. and G.

Late Dr. John Dicks, of Mid Calder (letter). 1885, 2, 231.

The case of Dr. David Bradley (letter). 1885, 2, 265.

On the treatment of acute peritonitis by abdominal section (letter). 1885, 1, 398.

The operative treatment of extra peritoneal peri-uterine haematoma (letter). 1885, 1, 699.

Kraurosis (abstract). 1875, 2, 59.

A new phase of Listerism. 1885, 2, 165.

–Edinburgh Med. J.

Note on chronic inflammatory disease of uterine appendages. 1885, 31, 201.

–Brit. Med. J.

The revival of ovariotomy (letter). 1885, 1, 49.

On one thousand abdominal sections. 1885, 1, 218.

Notes on cholecystotomy. 1885, 1, 275.

Note on three cases of tubal pregnancy successfully operated upon at the period of rupture. 1885, 1, 778.

Saccular dilatation of the urethra. 1885, 1, 982.

The modern treatment of uterine myoma. 1885, 2, 287.

Treatment of uterine myoma by removal of the appendages (letters). 1885, 2, 365, 416, 570 and 620.

A case of hysterectomy in which removal of the appendages had failed to arrest the haemorrhage or growth of the tumour. 1885, 2, 645.

On ligature in ovariotomy (letter). 1885, 2, 937.

Perinaeorraphy (letters). 1885, 2, 996 and 1183.

Nine cases of successful operations for ruptured tubal pregnancy. 1885, 2, 1158.

–Lancet.

Treatment of acute peritonitis by abdominal section (letter). 1885, 1, 1102.

The occurrence of jaundice as a symptom of gall-stone (letter). 1885, 2, 41.

The surgical treatment of gall-stones. 1885, 2, 379 and 422.

Vicarious menstruation (letter). 1885, 2, 690.

Case of inversion of the uterus (letter). 1885, 2, 877.

–Birm. Phil. Soc. Trans.

Progress of doctrine of evolution. 1885, 5, 1.

1885 (cont'd.)

–Med. Press and C.

A series of one thousand cases of abdominal section. 1885, 1, 65 and 89.

The report of experiments on living animals (letters). 1885, 2, 43 and 63.

Dr. Bradley's case (letter). 1885, 2, 242.

–Canadian Medical and Surgical Journal

Removal of the uterine appendages. 1885, 2, 77.

1886

–Edin. Med. J.

Diseases and removal of the uterine appendages (abstract). 1885-1886, 31, 812.

Inaugural address to the Wolverhampton Medical Society (Common-sense in the practice of Medicine). 1886-1887, 32, 481.

–Brit. Med. J.

The ligature in ovariotomy. 1886, 1, 229.

On abdominal section (abstract). 1886, 1, 413.

Pelvic haematocele (letter). 1886, 1, 523.

One hundred and thirty-nine consecutive ovariotomies performed between January 1st. 1884 and December 31st 1885 without a death. 1886, 1, 921.

Peritoneal surgery (letter). 1886, 1, 1042.

The revival of ovariotomy and Mr. Tait (letter). 1886, 1, 1196 and 2, 49.

Abstract of a paper on the general principles involved in the operation of removal of the uterine appendages. 1886, 2, 853.

On the surgical treatment of diseases of the liver. 1886, 2, 905.

An address on removal of the uterine appendages. 1886, 2, 1082.

–Lancet.

Five additional cases of cholecystotomy. 1886, 1, 296.

Use of iodide of potassium in aneurysm (letter). 1886, 1, 431.

An improvement in Paquelin's cautery (letter). 1886, 1, 998.

Four cases of chronic inflammatory disease of the uterine appendages. 1886, 2, 67.

Casey v. Imlach (letter). 1886, 2, 375.

Haematocele, intra- or extra- peritoneal (letters). 1886, 2, 470 and 653.

Spaying or removal of the uterine appendages (letter). 1886, 2, 557.

Hospital for Women, Liverpool (letter). 1886, 2, 796.

Ingleby lecture on pelvic haematocele. 1886, 2, 805.

General principles involved in the operation of removal of the uterine appendages (abstract). 1886, 2, 869.

Case of menstruation after removal of pregnant uterus and appendages. 1886, 2, 1173.

–Birm. Med. R.

Inaugural Address to the British Gynaecological Society. 1886, 19, 97.

–Med. Press and C.

Ingleby Lecture on abdominal surgery. 1886, 2, 421 and 455.

–Amer. J. Obst.

Oophorectomy in uterine fibroids (letter). 1886, 19, 483.

Abdominal section for pelvic abscess (letter). 1886, 19, 971.

1886 (cont'd.)

(–Amer. J. Obst.)

Methods of diagnosis (abstract). 1886, 19, 316.

Statistics of hysterectomy (letter). 1886, 19, 824.

Tait on Faradism (letter). 1886, 19, 1087.

The diagnosis of disease of the uterine appendages and the indications for Tait's operation (letter). 1886, 19, 1162.

–British Gynaecological Journal.

On some pending questions in gynaecology. 1886, 2, 19.

An address on the work and progress of the British Gynaecological Society. 1886, 2, 517.

–New York Med. J.

Chronic inflammatory disease of the uterine appendages (letters) 1886, 1, 699 and 2, 270.

A discussion of the general principles involved in the operation of removal of the uterine appendages. 1886, 2, 561.

–Provincial Medical Journal.

Methods of diagnosis. 1886, 5, 242.

–Practitioner.

Climacteric diabetes in women. 1886, 36, 401.

1887

–Brit. Med. J.

The Liverpool Hospital for Women (letter). 1887, 1, 303.

Dr. Skene Keith's statistics of abdominal surgery (letter). 1887, 1, 354, 481, 592 and 697.

Note on the pathology of chronic disease of the uterine appendages, as illustrated by the preparations of sixty-three cases removed during the year 1886. 1887, 1, 825.

The mortality after laparotomy for extra-uterine pregnancy (letters). 1887, 1, 747 and 907.

On the unsatisfactory results of unilateral removal of the uterine appendages. 1887, 1, 1211.

An address on the development of surgery and the germ theory. 1887, 2, 166.

On the treatment of uterine tumours by electricity (letters). 1887, 2, 964, 1075 and 1182.

Dr. Keith's remarks concerning the methods of treatment of uterine tumours (letter). 1887, 2, 1359.

–Lancet.

Note on hysterectomy. 1887, 1, 18.

The term "spaying" (letter). 1887, 1, 238.

The mere presence of blood in the peritoneal cavity not a reason for abdominal section (letters). 1887, 1, 290 and 397.

Pathology of tubal pregnancy (abstract). 1887, 1, 525.

The purgative treatment of peritonitis (letter) 1887, 2, 836.

The treatment of intestinal obstruction due to an impacted gall-stone (letter). 1887, 2, 1192.

A case of hystero-epilepsy successfully treated by removal of damaged uterine appendages. 1887, 2, 1213.

1887 (cont'd.)

–New York Med. J.

The germ theory and advances in abdominal surgery. 1887, 2, 1.

–Amer. J. Obst.

Early diagnosis of extra-uterine pregnancy (letter). 1887, 20, 515.

On the results of unilateral removal of the uterine appendages. 1887, 20, 478.

–Brit. Gyn. J.

Methods of cleansing the peritoneum. 1887, 3, 185.

On the method of flap-splitting in certain plastic operations. 1887, 3, 367.

Twelve cases of ruptured tubal pregnancy. 1887, 3, 415.

–Prov. Med. J.

A discussion of the general principles involved in the operation of removal of the uterine appendages. 1887, 6, 2.

Dr. Purcell's case of colpo-hysterectomy for malignant disease of the uterus (letter). 1887, 6, 575.

1888

–Brit. Med. J.

The electrical treatment of uterine tumours (letters). 1888, 1, 493 and 1085.

Menstruation after hysterectomy (letter). 1888, 1, 666.

A case in which ruptured tubal pregnancy occurred twice in the same patient. 1888, 1, 1001.

Urticaria diffusa occurring after ovariectomy (letter). 1888, 1, 1248.

Ectopic gestation (letter). 1888, 1, 1299.

The influence of removal of the uterus and its appendages on the sexual appetite (abstract). 1888, 1, 1387.

Pyosalpinx or suppurating parovarian cyst (letter). 1888, 2, 1023.

General summary of conclusions from a second series of one thousand consecutive cases of abdominal section. 1888, 2, 1096.

The antiseptic vaults at St. Mechans (letter). 1888, 2, 1416.

–Lancet.

Additional series of eleven cases of cholecystotomy. 1888, 1, 717.

Ovariotomy (letter). 1888, 2, 137.

Lecture on a case of ruptured tubal pregnancy. 1888, 2, 409.

Menstruation and the ovaries (letters). 1888, 2, 1044 and 1204.

Examination for the Fellowship of the Royal College of Surgeons (letter). 1888, 2, 1256.

–Birm. Med. R.

Introductory lecture to the class of Gynaecology in Queen's College, Birmingham. 1888, 24, 97.

–Med. Press and C.

A case of pyosalpinx. 1888, 1, 56.

–Amer. J. Obst.

Primary laparotomy in extra-uterine pregnancy by Dr. P. Harris. Note on extra-uterine pregnancy (letter). 1888, 21, 394.

Primary laparotomy in extra-uterine pregnancy. 1888, 21, 494.

A criticism and reply. 1888, 21, 289.

1888 (cont'd.)

–Brit. Gyn. J.

A research into the coincidence of ovulation and menstruation. 1888, 4, 89.

Note on the influence of removal of the uterus and its appendages on the sexual appetite. 1888, 4, 310.

–Prov. Med. J.

Lectures on Gynaecology: I Malformations. 1888, 7, 290.

Lectures on Gynaecology: II. 1888, 7, 338.

–Dublin Journal of Medical Science.

Note on the principle of flap splitting in plastic operations: A recognition of priority on the part of the late Maurice Collis. 1888, 1, 381.

–Medical News.

Masturbation. A clinical lecture. 1888, 53, 2.

–Pamphlets.

Criticism of doctrine of individuality. 1888. Birmingham.

Report of Mr. Councillor Lawson Tait and the M.O.H. upon the question of preparing a disease map of the Borough. 1888. Birmingham.

1889

–Edin. Med. J.

The pathological importance of the broad ligaments. 1889-1890, 35, 1 and 97.

The surgery of the liver. 1889, 35, 305 and 401.

–Brit. Med. J.

The College of Surgeons and its Members (letters). 1889, 1, 561, 915 and 1143.

The election of the College of Surgeons (letter). 1889, 1, 1322 and 2, 154.

Clinical lecture on uterine myoma. 1889, 2, 299.

The Royal College of Surgeons and its bye-laws (letter). 1889, 2, 338.

Insanity following surgical operations (letter). 1889, 2, 497.

Case of recurrent perityphlitis successfully treated by abdominal section. 1889, 2, 763.

Renal surgery. 1889, 2, 1085.

–Lancet.

Reform at the Royal College of Surgeons (letters). 1889, 1, 97, 448, 653 and 809.

Ectopic pregnancy and pelvic haematocele (letter). 1889, 1, 193.

Note on a case of cholecystotomy. 1889, 1, 1294.

The recent election at the Royal College of Surgeons (letter). 1889, 2, 137.

Ectopic pregnancy (letter). 1889, 2, 458.

A case of intraperitoneal haematocele due to rupture of a tubal pregnancy treated by abdominal section and removal of the ruptured tube. 1889, 2, 1054.

–Med. Press and C.

Ectopic gestation. 1889, 2, 375.

–Amer. J. Obst.

Tait vs. Morrel on ruptured tubal pregnancy. 1889, 22, 400.

The flap-splitting operation for lacerated perineum (letter). 1889, 22, 1044.

1889 (cont'd.)

–Brit. Gyn. J.
A criticism of some recent utterances on ectopic gestation. 1889, 5, 454.
–Prov. Med. J.
On ectopic gestation. 1889, 8, 645.

1890

–Brit. Med. J.
The "Porro-Caesarean" operation (letters). 1890, 1, 154 and 573.
An address on the surgical aspect of impacted labour. 1890, 1, 657.
The surgical treatment of impacted labour (letter). 1890, 1, 864.
Mistakes concerning ectopic gestation (letter). 1890, 1, 924.
The present position of abdominal surgery (abstract). 1890, 1, 955.
Ectopic pregnancy in the broad ligament (letter). 1890, 1, 1044.
The discussion at the Medical Society on abdominal surgery (letters). 1890, 1, 1105 and 1219.
The election at the College of Surgeons (letter). 1890, 2, 113.
Address in Surgery. Surgical training, surgical practice. Surgical results. 1890, 2, 267.
An address on the present aspect of antiseptic surgery. 1890, 2, 728.
Scepticism and asepticism (letter). 1890, 2, 925 and 1092.
The surgical treatment of uterine myoma. 1890, 2, 1005.
The treatment of uterine myoma (letters). 1890, 2, 1149, 1272 and 1600.
–Lancet.
The recent election to the College of Surgeons (letter). 1890, 1, 94.
The after history of a case of Caesarean Section. 1890, 2, 766.
Abdominal surgery (letter). 1890, 2, 997.
The Royal College of Surgeons (letters). 1890, 2, 1056, 1136 and 1248.
–Birm. Med. R.
The surgical treatment of typhilitis. 1890, 27, 26 and 76.
–Med. P. and C.
Indications for abdominal section and the details of its performance. 1890, 1, 369.
A contribution to the debate on the present position of abdominal surgery. 1890, 1, 419.
The discussion at the Medical Society on abdominal surgery (letter). 1890, 1, 489.
Hysterectomy and electrolysis for uterine myomata (letter). 1890, 2, 483.
The treatment of uterine myoma (letters). 1890, 2, 618 and 700.
–Prov. Med. J.
A criticism of some recent utterances on ectopic gestation. 1890, 9, 194.

1891

–Brit. Med. J.
The treatment of uterine myoma (letter). 1891, 1, 87.

1891 (cont'd.)

(–Brit. Med. J.)

Recent debates on gynaecology (letter). 1891, 1, 199.

Practical cure or disastrous failure (letter). 1891, 1, 316.

The present position of antiseptic surgery (letter). 1891, 1, 381.

The treatment of tumours by electricity (letter). 1891, 1, 609.

A discussion on treatment of hernia by median abdominal section. 1891, 2, 685.

The modern treatment of uterine myoma (letter). 1891, 2, 1022.

–Lancet.

Recent debates on gynaecology (letter). 1891, 1, 221.

Address on the principle of exploratory and confirmatory incisions. 1891, 1, 292.

Failure or cure? (letter). 1891, 1, 338.

Sequel to a case of abdominal section (letters). 1891, 1, 1067 and 1228.

Treatment of chronic inflammatory disease of the uterine appendages (letters). 1891, 1, 573 and 849.

The recent election at the College of Surgeons (letters). 1891, 2, 146 and 406.

Clinical lecture on the details necessary in the performance of abdominal section. 1891, 2, 597.

The use of antiseptics (letters). 1891, 2, 843, 896, 956, 1013 and 1068.

–Med. Press and C.

An address on the remote effects of removal of the uterine appendages. 1891, 1, 367.

Repair of the female perineum. 1891, 2, 25.

–Prov. Med. J.

Electrical treatment of uterine tumours (letter). 1891, 10, 384.

1892

–Brit. Med. J.

The Medical Defence Union (letter). 1892, 1, 145.

The modern treatment of uterine myoma (letter). 1892, 1, 197.

Female Inebriety (letter). 1892, 2, 871.

The total abolition and suppression of vivisection (abstract). 1892, 2, 1024.

Mr. Tait and antivivisection (letters). 1892, 2, 1032 and 1139.

Peritonitis: its nature and prevention. 1892, 2, 1046.

The treatment of peritonitis (letter). 1892, 2, 1198.

Mr. Tait and the Scientific Grants Committee (letter). 1892, 2, 1365.

–Lancet.

The corpus luteum (letter). 1892, 1, 56.

Uterine dilatation (letter). 1892, 1, 1000.

The Council of the Royal College of Surgeons (letter). 1892, 1, 1053, 1271 and 1385.

Alleged occcurrence of ovarian pregnancy (abstract). 1892, 1, 1364.

Experiments upon animals (setters). 1892, 2, 1138, 1302 and 1468.

1892 (cont'd.)

–Lancet.

A case of ectopic pregnancy in which the foetus seems to have been developed to the full time in the peritoneal cavity, still retaining its amniotic covering. 1892, 34, 192.

Two cases of hysterectomy. 1892, 34, 199.

Notes on the growth of the placenta after death of the foetus in ectopic gestation (with Christopher Martin). 1892, 34, 199.

–Med. Chir. Trans.

On the occurrence of pleural effusion in association with disease of the abdomen. 1892, 75, 109.

Note on the alleged occurrence of ovarian pregnancy. 1892, 75, 387.

–Med. Press and C.

Notes on the alleged occurrence of tubal abortion. 1892, 1, 285.

–Prov. Med. J.

Peritonitis. Its nature and prevention. 1892, 11, 641.

1893

–Brit. Med. J.

The end of a practical cure (letter). 1893, 1, 546.

–Lancet.

The sensitiveness of the peritoneum. 1893, 1, 125.

The sensitiveness of the peritoneum (letters). 1893, 1, 273 and 447.

British Institute of Preventive Medicine (letters). 1893, 1, 388 and 497.

A simple method of performing suprapubic cystostomy. 1893, 1, 1254.

A case of nephrorrhaphy. 1893, 2, 1281.

–Med. Press.

Ectopic gestation. 1893, 1, 506.

–Prov. Med. J.

A clinical lecture on the diagnosis of pregnancy. 1893, 12, 397, 476, and 535.

1894

–Brit. Med. J.

The late Dr. Charles Clay of Manchester (letter). 1894, 1, 1278.

Septic catheters (letter). 1894, 1, 1413.

–Lancet.

A case of interstitial pregnancy successfully treated by abdominal section. 1894, 1, 88.

The ethics of hospitals (letter). 1894, 2, 463.

The Women's Free Hospital, Southampton (letter). 1894, 2, 1133.

–Birm. Med. R.

Notes on anaesthetics. 1894, 35, 285.

–Med. Press and C.

A criticism of the germ theory of disease. 1894, 2, 476.

1894 (cont'd.)

–Prov. Med. J.

Vivisection (letter). 1894, 13, 223.

An analysis of the evidence in seventy consecutive cases of changes made under the new Criminal Law Amendment Act. 1894, 13, 226.

A criticism of the "Germ theory of Disease based on the Baconian method". 1894, 13, 567.

1895

–Brit. Med. J.

A question of conscience (letter). 1895, 2, 870.

–Lancet.

The Women's Free Hospital, Southampton (letters). 1895, 1, 893 and 1144.

Perforation of uterus by sound or curette. 1895, 2, 327.

Note on a rare condition of the omentum (letter). 1895, 2, 428.

Over-operating in gynaecology (letters). 1895, 2, 755 and 941.

–Med. Press and C.

The dangers of secondary haemorrhage from a broad ligament pedicle and the best preventative. 1895, 2, 1.

–Prov. Med. J.

Note on the processes of menstruation. 1895, 14, 6.

Mr. Lawson Tait's paper on the Germ Theory (letter). 1895, 14, 55.

–Brit. Med. J.

The advance of abdominal surgery (letter). 1896, 1, 629.

–Lancet.

Metro-peritoneal fistula in a criminal prosecution (letter). 1896, 1, 325.

A new electrical haemostat (abstract). 1896, 1, 781.

The evolution of the surgical treatment of the broad ligament pedicle. 1896, 1, 1338.

The evolution of the surgical treatment of the broad ligament pedicle (letter). 1896, 1, 1456.

Thomas Keith and the cautery (letter). 1896, 2, 52.

The possibility of ovarian pregnancy (letter). 1896, 2, 493.

An acoustic bladder sound and vaginal stethoscope (letter). 1896, 2, 1558.

–Med. Press and C.

Cleansing and cleanliness in abdominal surgery. 1896, 2, 539 and 569.

1897

–Brit. Med. J.

The treatment of myoma (letter). 1897, 1, 301.

Robert Houston's ovariotomy, 1701 (letter). 1897, 1, 559.

The modern treatment of myomatous disease of the uterus. 1897, 1, 779.

Tait's flap-splitting operation on the perineum (letter). 1897, 2, 1298.

1897 (cont'd.)

–Lancet.

The treatment of myoma (letter). 1897, 1, 405.

An unusual case of tubal abortion (letter). 1897, 1, 623.

A question for anaesthetists (letter). 1897, 1, 988.

A new pattern of scissors for perineal repair. 1897, 1, 1216.

The question of the second ovary in ovariotomy (letter). 1897, 1, 1236.

Excision of parovarian cysts without removal of the tube (letter). 1897, 1, 1502.

The late Dr. Braxton Hicks (letter). 1897, 2, 744.

A question of title (letter). 1897, 2, 1483.

–Birm. Med. R.

Was Robert Houston, of Glasgow, the first ovariotomist?1897. 41, 277.

1898

–Brit. Med. J.

Anaesthetics (letter). 1898, 1, 919.

The etiology of typhus fever (letter). 1898, 1, 1047.

A new and original method of making casts (letter). 1898, 2, 748.

–Lancet.

The unqualified assistant and the General Medical Council (letters). 1898, 1, 328 and 466.

A method of exposing and operating on the kidney without division of muscles, vessels or nerves (letter). 1898, 1, 1428.

Note on lumbar colotomy. 1898, 1, 1747.

A physical basis in the drunkenness of women (letter). 1898, 2, 227.

The so-called conservative surgery of the uterine appendages (letter). 1898, 2, 778.

–Amer. J. Obst.

Statistics of abdominal section in America (letter). 1898, 1, 624.

–Med. Press and C.

The evolution of the aseptic method in surgery. 1898, 1, 427.

1899

–Brit. Med. J.

The Causa Causans of typhus fever (letter). 1899, 1, 879.

A charge against the Chairman of Council (letter). 1899, 1, 1439.

–Lancet.

On the treatment of "unavoidable haemorrhage" by removal of the uterus. 1899, 1, 364.

–Birm. Med. R.

The bedstead as an important factor in domestic hygiene and comfort. 1899, 45, 257.

–Med. Press and C.

The term "Conservative Surgery" as it has been proposed to apply it to the uterus and its appendages. 1899, 1, 341.

III. BOOKS AND MONOGRAPHS

1874

Compendium of Children's Diseases. Johann Steiner. (Trans. Lawson Tait). 1874. Churchill, London.

The Pathology and Treatment of Diseases of the Ovary, Being the Hasting's Prize Essay of 1873. Lawson Tait. 1874. Smith Elder, London.

1877

Diseases of Women. Lawson Tait. 1877. Williams and Norgate, London.

An Essay on Hospital Mortality Based upon the Statistics of Hospitals of Great Britain for Fifteen Years. Lawson Tait. 1877. Birmingham.

1879

Diseases of Women. Lawson Tait. 1879. Ward, New York.

1883

Diseases of the Ovaries. Lawson Tait. 1883. Cornish Bros., Birmingham and New York.

The Pathology and Treatment of Diseases of the Ovaries. Lawson Tait. 1883. Cornish Bros., Birmingham and New York.

1886

Traité des maladies des ovaires suivi d'une étude sur quelques progrès récents de la chirurgie abdominale et pelvienne. Lawson Tait. 1886. (Trans. by Dr. Oliver. Paris.

1889

Diseases of Women and Abdominal Surgery. Lawson Tait. Vol. I. 1889. Richardson, Leicester and Lea Bros., Philadelphia.

1891

Traité clinique des maladies des femmes. Lawson Tait. (Trans. by Albert Bétrix). 1891. Paris.

INDEX OF PERSONAL NAMES

Note: Practitioners of medicine, whatever their qualifications or titles, are listed by surname and initials. (In a few cases the surname only has been given.) The differentiation Mr. or Dr., indicating surgeon or physician, is ignored as this did not come into strict use until after 1900. Women doctors are listed by surname and forename. Those other than practitioners of medicine are listed by surname followed by Mr., Mrs., Miss, Rev., Prof., Sir etc. (Additional names occurring in the references are not indexed).

. . . .

GENERAL INDEX

Note: Surgical and medical references are limited to major topics arising in the text. Frequent minor references to Birmingham, Edinburgh and London are not listed.

. . . .

ILLUSTRATIONS

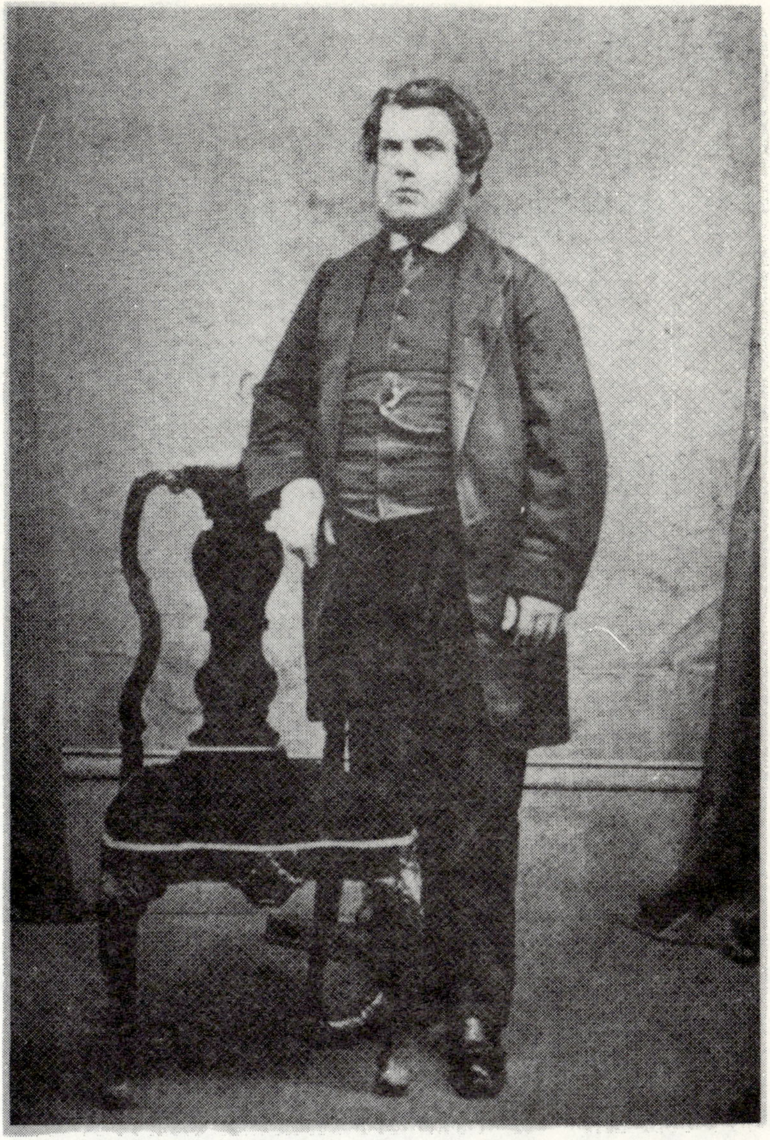

III Tait as a Student (c. 1866)

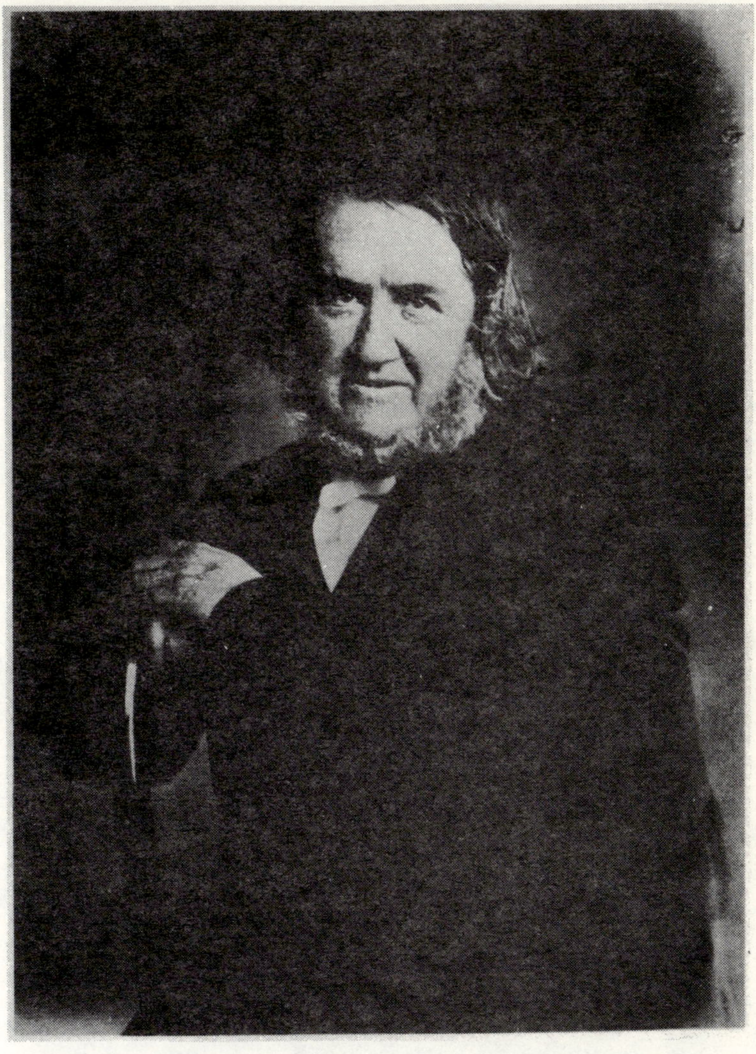

IV Sir James Young Simpson (c. 1867)
(By permission of the Librarian of St. Andrews University)

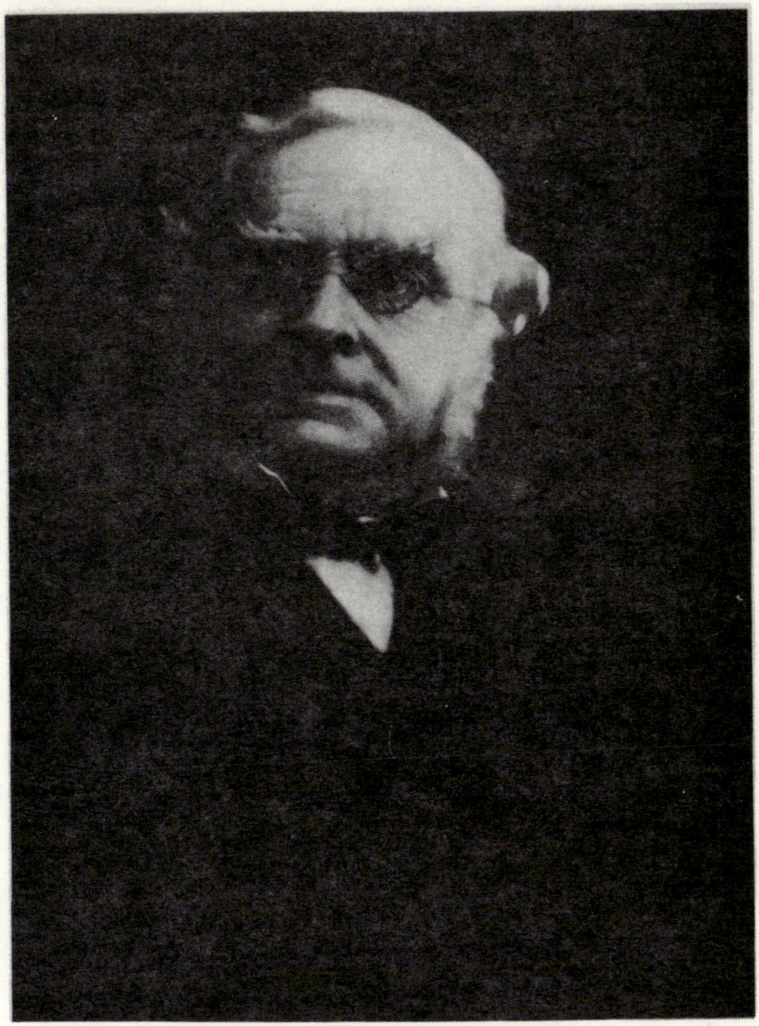

V Sir Thomas Spencer Wells (c. 1885)
(By permission of the Royal College
of Obstetricians and Cynaecologists)

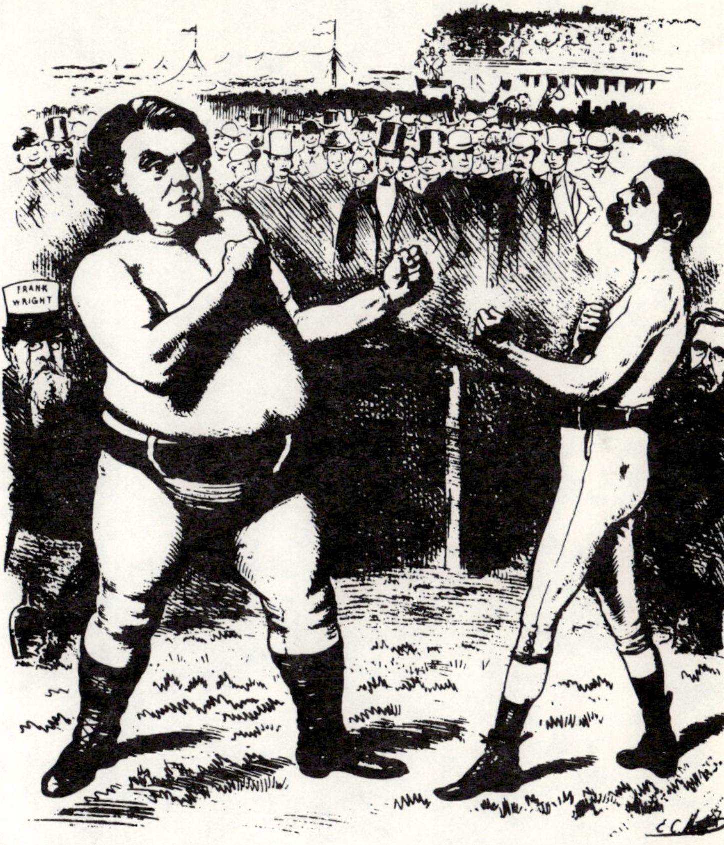

VI Political Cartoon. Tait sparring with Randolph Churchill
(From a Birmingham Paper *The Dart*, 1887)

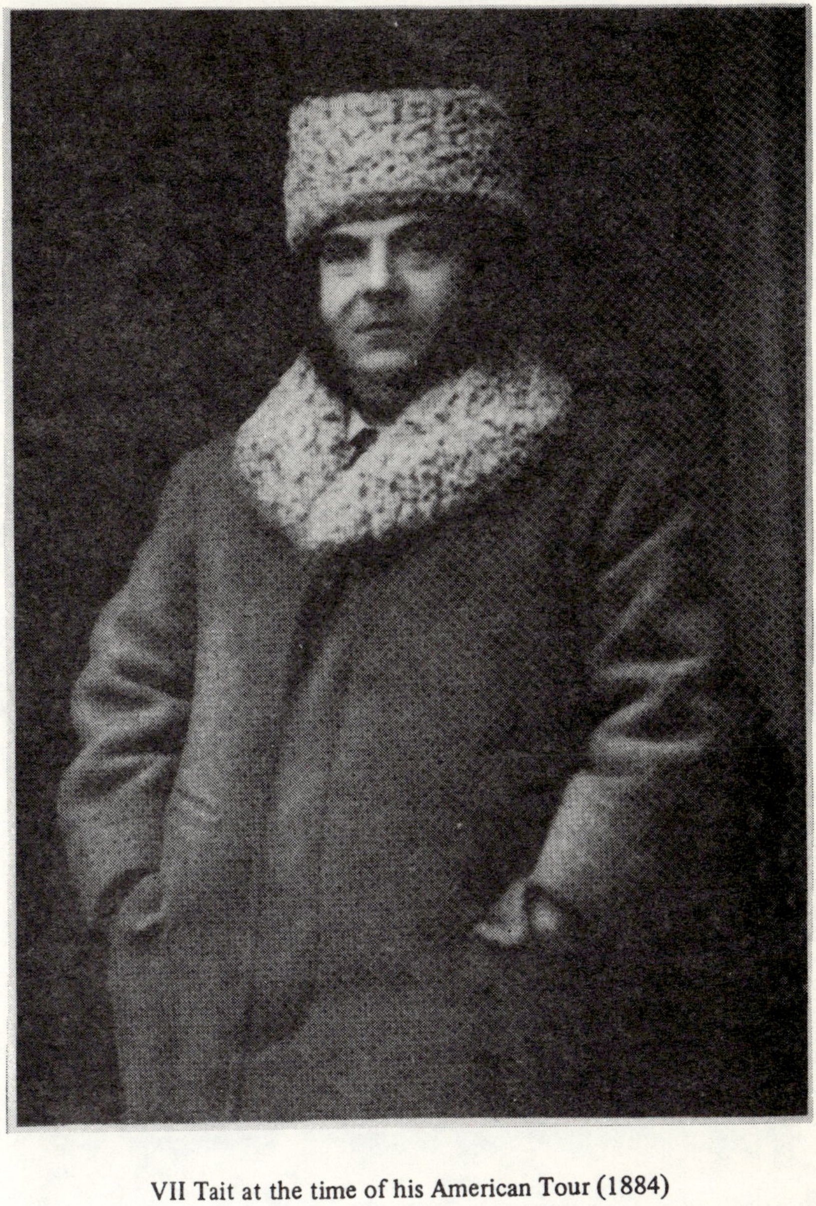

VII Tait at the time of his American Tour (1884)

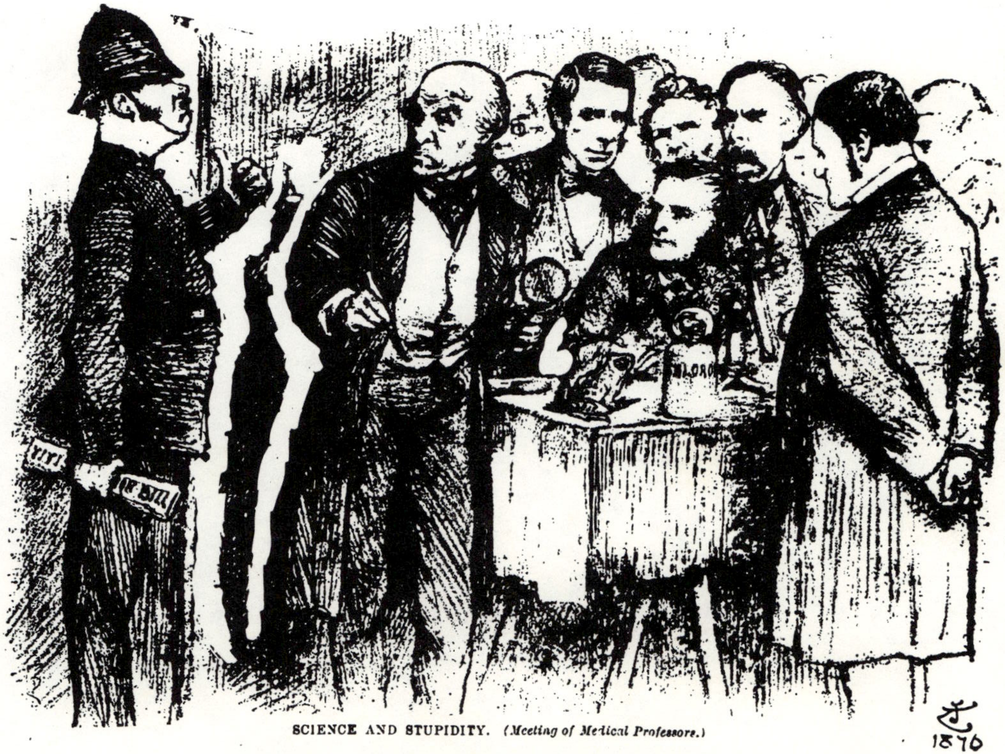

SCIENCE AND STUPIDITY. *(Meeting of Medical Professors.)*

VIII Cartoon with pro-vivisectionists Drs. Jenner, Paget, Hart and Gull (By permission of the proprietors of *Punch*)

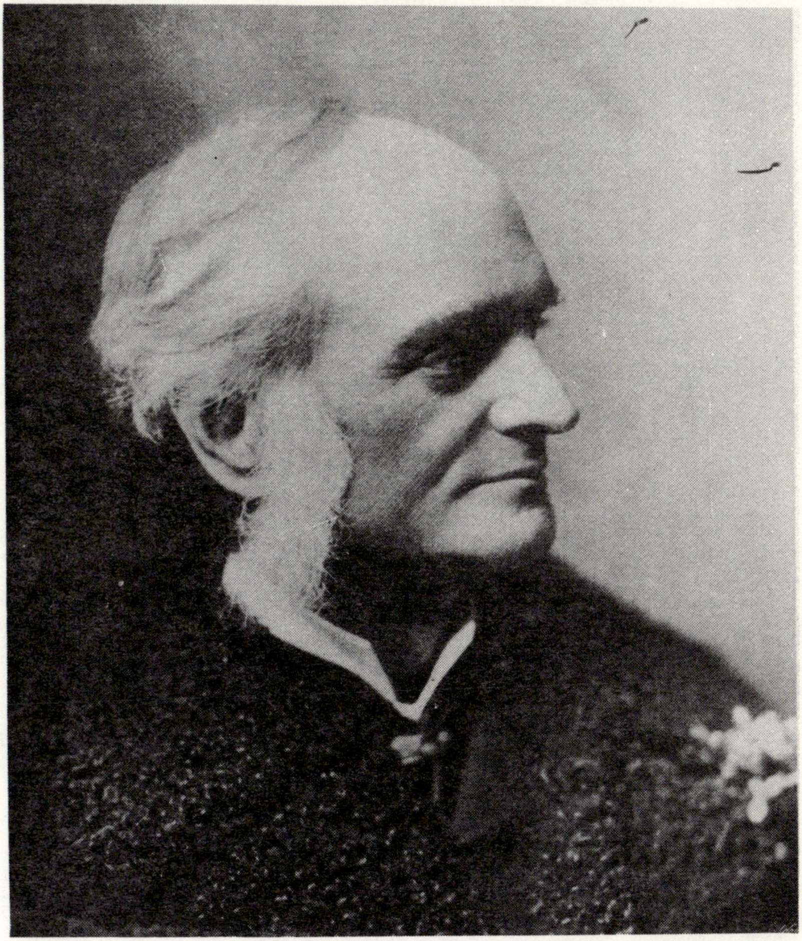

IX Dr. Ernest Hart (1835-1898)

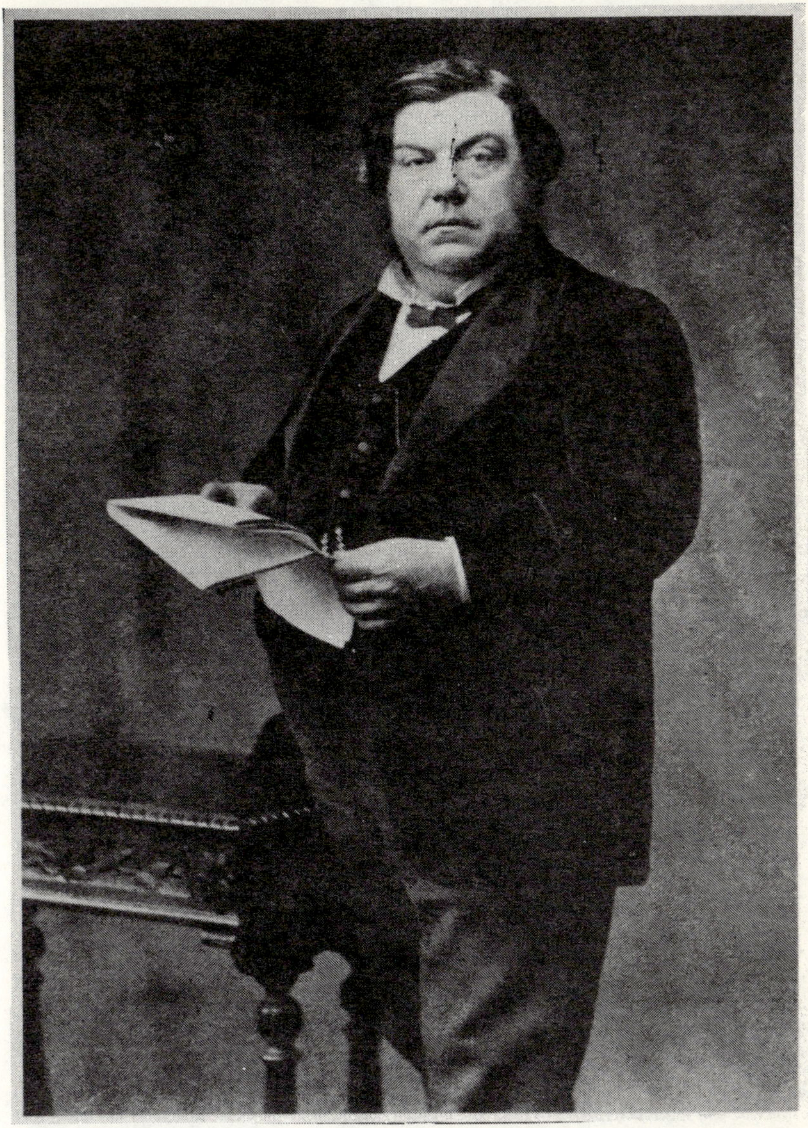

X Lawson Tait (1890)

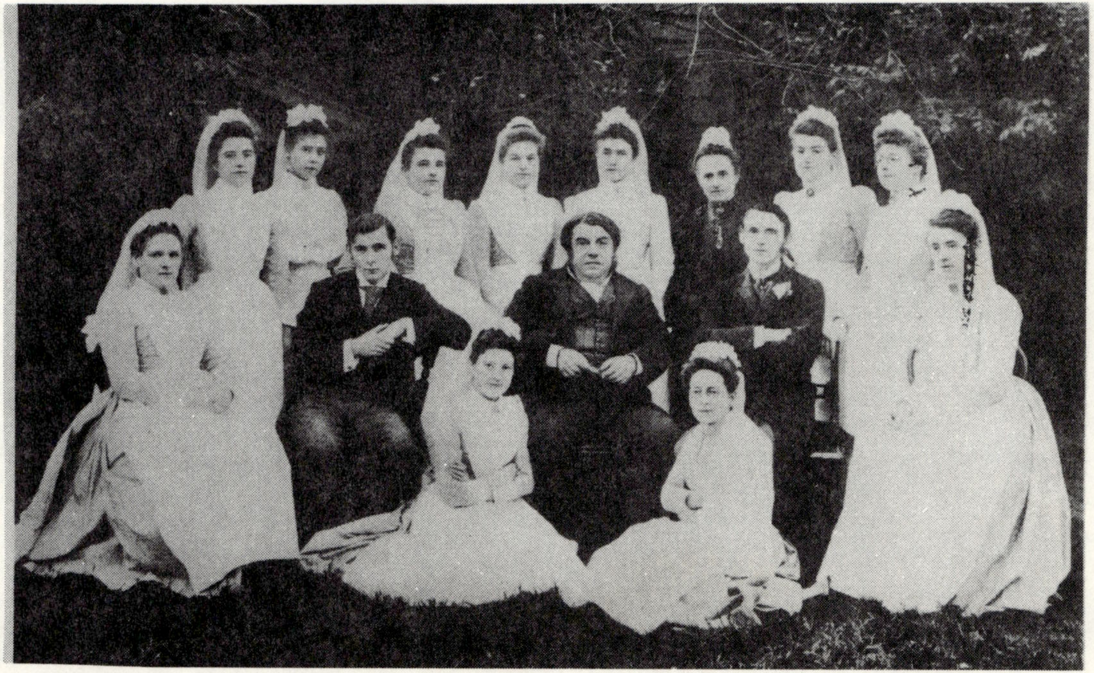

XI Tait and his staff at the Crescent (c. 1891). Christopher Martin, his assistant is on Tait's left. Charles Martin, his secretary, is on Tait's right

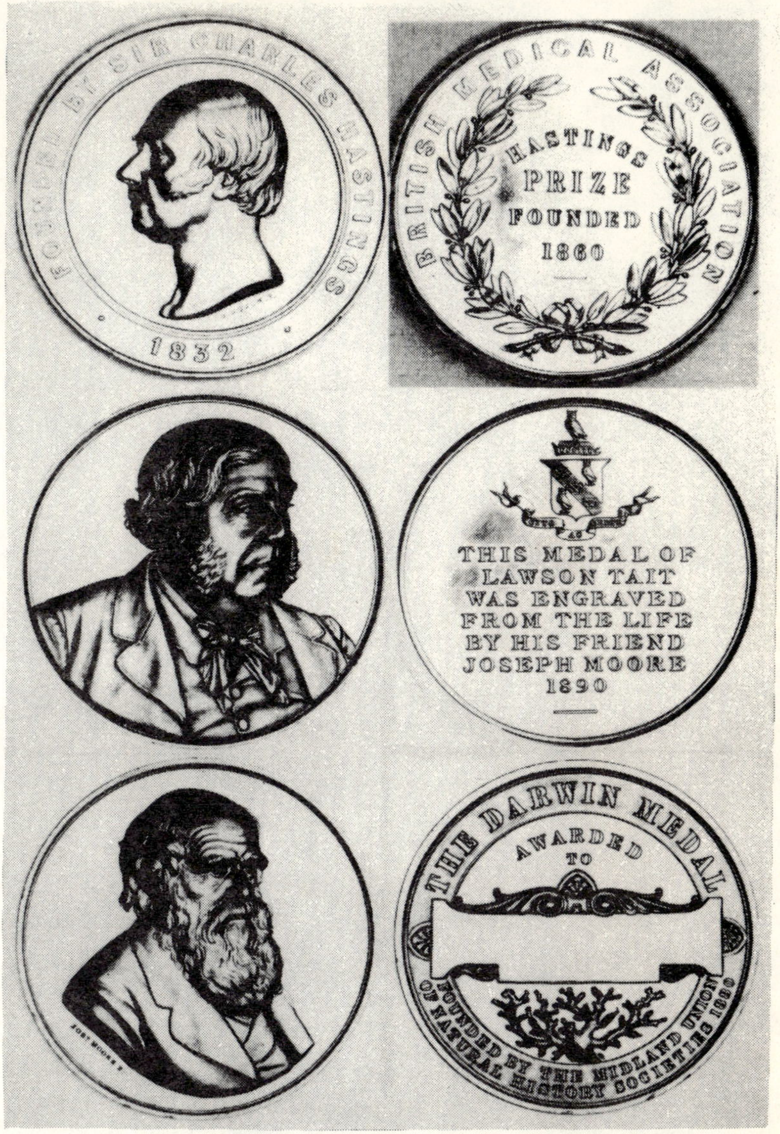
FOUNDED BY SIR CHARLES HASTINGS
1832
BRITISH MEDICAL ASSOCIATION
HASTINGS
PRIZE
FOUNDED
1860
THIS MEDAL OF
LAWSON TAIT
WAS ENGRAVED
FROM THE LIFE
BY HIS FRIEND
JOSEPH MOORE
1890
THE DARWIN MEDAL
AWARDED
TO
FOUNDED BY THE MIDLAND UNION
OF NATURAL HISTORY SOCIETIES 1880

XII Top: Hastings Gold Medal awarded to Tait

Middle: Bronze medal of Tait

Foot: Bronze medal of Charles Darwin